Praise

Look Out Cancer Here I Come!

"This is the insightful and inspirational story of a remarkable survivor. Many patients and their physicians could benefit from her experience, her wisdom and her spirit."

—Robert C. Bast, Jr., M.D.
VP Translational Research
M.D. Anderson Cancer Center

"An inspirational book for anyone with cancer or other illnesses. Sharon captures the feelings patients experience and outlines a positive approach to coping. Essential reading for both men and women who find themselves diagnosed with a serious illness."

—Robert A Press, M.D., Ph.D.
Clinical Associate Professor of Medicine
NYU School of Medicine

"This entertaining book reads like a novel, but is totally based on facts. It will both comfort and empower you. If you are being treated for cancer, you should refer to it repeatedly throughout your treatment for a quick uplift of the spirit and a lot of humor and love."

—Ruth L. Katz M.D.
Chief Research Cytopathology
M.D. Anderson Cancer Center

"Sharon Parker captures the essence of a cancer patient's journey from discovery of the disease to its cure. Her book is a must read for cancer patients, families, and treating professionals."

—Andrew L. Pecora, MD F.A.C.P
Chairman and Executive Administrative Director
The Cancer Center at Hackensack University Medical Center

Look Out Cancer Here I Come!

*How I Beat the Odds
and Came Out a Winner*

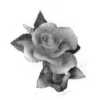

Sharon Lee Parker

Addicus Books
Omaha, Nebraska

An Addicus Nonfiction Book

10-ISBN: 1-886039-10-0
13-ISBN: 978-1-886039-1-00
Cover design by Peri Poloni
Cover photo by Robin Roslund, Boca Raton, FL
The porcelain "Hope Rose," shown on the cover, is produced by the Boehm Porcelain Company.

The opinions put forth in this book are solely those of the author, based on her personal experience. This book is not intended to serve as a substitute for a physician. Nor is it the author's intent to give medical advice contrary to that of an attending physician.

Library of Congress Cataloging-in-Publication Data

Parker, Sharon L.
    Look out cancer, here I come : how I beat the odds and came out a winner / Sharon Lee Parker.
        p. cm.
    "An Addicus nonfiction book."
    10-ISBN: 1-886039-10-0; 13-ISBN: 978-1-886039-1-00 (alk. paper)
    1. Parker, Sharon L.--Health. 2. Hodgkin's disease–Patients--United States--Biography. I. Title.
    RC644.P37 2006
    362.196'994460092--dc22
B   2005025959

Addicus Books, Inc.
P.O. Box 45327
Omaha, Nebraska 68145
www.AddicusBooks.com

Printed in the United States of America
10 9 8 7 6 5 4 3 2 1

To all the mothers, fathers, husbands, wives, sons, daughters, caregivers, friends, and researchers who make a profound difference in the quality of life of every cancer patient; and to the doctors, nurses, and hospital staff who help us focus on a positive outlook and a bright tomorrow.

In Honor of
Cecilia R. Strauss

January 13, 1916—September 19, 2002

My extraordinary mother died after an unexpected bout with cancer just shy of her eighty-seventh birthday in her hometown of Danby, Vermont; at the same time, I was undergoing chemotherapy in Houston, Texas.

A speech professor, she had the unique ability to share her wisdom and kindness with everyone she touched. Positive reinforcement was among her greatest strengths, and she lovingly encouraged friends, family, and total strangers to reach their fullest potential and loftiest goals.

"You are a wonder," she often said to her children, with a warmth that brings tears to my eyes. However, if anyone deserved that accolade, it was she without question.

Contents

Foreword

I first met Sharon Parker in April 2002 in my clinic at M.D. Anderson Cancer Center. I knew from our first encounter that she would take a very proactive role in her treatment. I confirmed this impression repeatedly throughout my association with her. Not only was she curious and questioning about the treatment we provided, but she also wanted to know what she should do herself to get better. She wanted to be an active part of her treatment, which I completely supported. I believe every patient is a crucial part of the team in his or her healing process.

What is remarkable in Sharon Parker's story is that she was dealing with multiple a diagnosis—Hodgkin's Disease and thyroid cancer. In her book, she not only tells this story, but draws from her experiences to offer recommendations to others—things they can do to cope when dealing with cancer.

Her outgoing personality and compassion came through while she was undergoing treatment; she would engage in conversation every step of the way with nurses, aides, clerks, technicians, and more importantly, other patients. In our waiting room, we observed her warmth and caring toward other patients. In medicine we call it the "human equation."

Sharon's courage and enthusiasm resonate throughout this book. Her message is clear: her active participation in her treatment made her feel better at every step along the way. She also helped herself by surrounding herself with supportive people. All this helped her overcome her fears.

Sharon's mission is now geared to supporting cancer research and volunteering to "coach" other cancer patients. Her mix of experience, compassion, and personality provide a unique combination that no doubt will help cancer patients and their loved ones.

—Andre Goy, M.D., M.S.
Chief of the Division of Lymphoma
The Cancer Center at Hackensack
University Medical Center

Acknowledgments

To George Parker, my husband, a computer wizard who was steadfast in helping bring this book to completion. To John Parker, my son, and Amy Sumida, my daughter, who encouraged me to stay focused and finish the task at hand.

To my publisher, Rod Colvin, of Addicus Books, for bringing this book to the forefront and making it available to so many readers. To Rudy Shur, of Square One Books, a distinguished mentor and advisor. To Lilly and Lawrence Wajnberg, who were impressed enough with the courage and information in the manuscript to publish it in Russian.

I know that I am here today, still on the road of life, because of Dr. André Goy. If I had to have cancer, God must have picked this brilliant oncologist and researcher to lead the team that would eradicate the lymphoma from my body. To Dr. Steven Sherman and Dr. Douglas Evans who monitor my thyroid for any changes. To the M.D. Anderson Cancer Center doctors and nurses who ensure that each patient who passes through the doors of their fabulous research hospital gets the best possible care. To Dr. Ruth Rheingold Katz, who introduced me to Houston at its best.

To Dr. Robert Press, who told me come to New York so that he could find out what was really wrong. Thank God, I followed my instincts.

To Richard Rubenstein, of Rubenstein Public Relations, who felt from the onset that the message the book imparts was important enough to bring it to the publics' eye. To television and radio personality Joe Franklin who has been steadfast in his determination to see this book in print.

To Arthur Redgrave, Norma Trusch and Paul Marshall, the attorneys who gave me sage advice and encouragement.

To my agent Arnold Graham, who never let me down and supported me through both the cancer treatment and writing this book.

A special thanks to Georgia and Congressman Benjamin Gilman whose warmth, wisdom and concern were ever-present.

To all my friends in Tuxedo Park, New York, and at St. Mary's Episcopal Church who had me on their prayer list every Sunday including Pamela and Ed Cromey, Serene and Phil Swirbul, Zosia and Penn Rogers, Glovina Schwartz, Sally and Chris Sonne, Elaine Romero, Manda and Mehrdad Sanandaji, Ed Wheeler, Adelaide Miller, Elizabeth (Betsy) Cathcart, Charlen and Jim Cathcart, Connie and John Vandenberg, Sistee and Richard Phillips, Mary Diem, and Gita May. I thank you for every good wish. To Judy and Dirk Salz whose e-mails were an inspiration of love which added to my determination to forge ahead.

To the Boehm Porcelain Company—Helen Boehm, Richard Vassil, and Maria Ristaino—your beautiful Hope Rose will inspire many to find a cure for Hodgkin's and non-Hodgkin's lymphoma. To the Concord Jewelers for their impeccable design of the, "I'm a Life Lover™" necklaces which are going to benefit the Life Lover™ Foundation, Inc.

To editor Claire Landiss for her creative ideas and fine research and to England's Dr. Michael Likosky who helped bring the manuscript to its finest state with unbridled enthusiasm.

To Dr. Gary Strauss, who said I could call at any time and, as a published medical writer and editor, agreed to read the manuscript. He flew from Chapel Hill, North Carolina, a few days before the arrival of the unwelcome Hurricane Francis, to proofread without the help of electricity; reminding us of the tenacity Abe Lincoln must have shown studying to become a lawyer in Illinois. As he kissed me good-bye, he said in earnest, "This is going to be a very important book for a lot of people. I think your father should read it."

To my father, Michael Strauss, who at age ninety-two, is still the sports editor of the *Palm Beach Daily News* in Florida and after seventy-five years in the newspaper business, he is still going strong. Sitting in my living room and gleaning over each word during the 2004 hurricanes, he made several poignant suggestions.

To Joe Scognamillo, Sal Scognamillo, and Frank DiCola, owners of Patsy's Italian Restaurant on West 56th Street in New York City, who believed in this book and encouraged me to continue from the first early draft right through to the published version.

To Horst and Anna Finkbeiner, Dr. William and Merry Likosky, and Charles and Evelyn Cathcart—your compassion and caring cannot be overstated.

To Patty and Al Carlson and Tom and Katie Magrann who want to eradicate cancer as much as I do.

To Harriet and Judge Burt Ledina whose joy of life will never be forgotten. To Susan and Paul Pashkow who couldn't wait for this book to come out. To Leiba and Neil Sedaka whose music, friendship and love have always been an important part of my life. To Sandy and Steven Richman who always knew what to say to keep my spirits high. To Ellen and Peter Boer, my sister and brother-in-law, who wanted nothing more than to have my cancer go away. To Paula and Bruce Merrifield and Rose and Larry Bauman for their inspiration and courage.

To Stephanie Parker for her undying support and encouragement. To Chrissy Parker and Aaron Sumida whose kind words and deeds are in my heart.

To my special friends from Florida for all their good wishes and inspiration: Alice and Andy Mossberg, Beverly and Larry Chaplin, June and Dr. Ira Gelb, Ellen Schaffer, Jaime and Howard Odzer, Eileen Carlson and Marilyn Forem. To Carol and Sidney Lerman who have been a tower of strength since they eloped in the early 1960s. To Pat Mistretta and Sandra Sicolo, my two Palm Beach County friends who encouraged me to finish this book, were kind enough to read the first manuscripts, and made some wonderful suggestions.

To my treasured aunts and uncles: Dorothy, Seymour, Auntie Mame, Ray, Gloria, and Jack Strauss. To Barbara, Richard, John, Nina, Cindy, and Pamela, thank you for helping me keep my mind focused and going in the right direction.

To all the doctors, nurses, clinicians, and friends who helped me heal and come out a winner: Drs. Francis Adams, Robert Bast, Alexa Kimball, Basil Chi-for, Robert Colvin, Bernard Crawford, Charles Debrovner, Elizabeth Hunsaker, Kenneth Hymes, Joan Minsky, Andrew Pecora, Mehrdad Sanandaji, Terry Simon, and Andrew Zelenetz.

My deepest gratitude to Marriott International and especially to Tye Turman and Debbie Bonafede for your gracious service and hospitality.

Lastly, to my little treasures, Amanda Grace, Andrea Claire, Matthew, and A. J. who give me nothing but joy and happiness every time I am lucky enough to see them.

Introduction

Racing through life was the name of the game.
I started to play it and was never the same.
Running here and running there,
No time to dream, no time to beware.

©Sharon Parker

Just like the little Nash Rambler, in the song "Beep
Beep," I was racing through life and couldn't stop. Remembering my life before cancer is like remembering a dream:
there are vivid impressions and memories, but now they
seem closer to a movie or even a cartoon than they do to
real life.

My life certainly maximizes that impression. At age six,
I was a competitive swimmer, racing round and round the
pool at the Women's Swimming Association on 23rd Street
in New York, trying to catch up with—or better, beat—my
sister Ellen. My father was a sportswriter for the *New York
Times*, and he was convinced that we were both on our way
to fame, fortune, and Olympic championship.

When those dreams didn't come true, new ones came
to take their place: I won a radio talent contest at age ten,
landed a record contract with Jubilee Records, and then
landed a bigger one with ABC Paramount. I was performing
every week, experiencing all the exhilaration of being on
stage as a young star, and was still finishing my homework
on time for high school. Sleep was little more than an annoying interruption of it all. The real dream happened when I
was awake.

Marrying George Parker—an heir to the Concord Hotel—at the tender age of nineteen put me in the fast lane permanently. I can still hear my mother-in-law whispering in my ear, "Remember, you married a hotel," as we prepared to make our vows in front of nine hundred guests I barely knew. Then, I had no idea what she meant, but I soon learned.

Standing in the middle of a dining room for three thousand, my job was to welcome as many vacationers as possible. Usually, I would circle the table in a fancy gown and spread my greetings as warmly as I could. As I finished with one table, I'd catch the eye of someone at another and begin my greetings there.

When Kenny Rogers, Neil Sedaka, Paul Anka, Tony Bennett, Joan Rivers, or any other celebrity arrived backstage at the Imperial Room, I offered a special welcome. Laden with fresh flowers and a personal note, I let each one know how much we appreciated his or her coming.

The first element that stands out in my life before cancer (and in ourselves as a culture) is plain busyness. As palm pilots, personal digital assistants (PDAs), cell phones, and a billion other devices keep us wired to the moment, it's increasingly easy to get into the habit of asking "what's next?" instead of "what's worth rushing to?" Even in this past decade, I have watched these trends become more pronounced, while the number of people being diagnosed with cancer keeps going up, up, up.

Like most people, I occasionally took time to reflect on the more important issues, but my primary focus was on today, tomorrow, and next week. Being high achievers, our family didn't block out any time for vacations or relaxing. The Concord was known as a *Titanic* on land, a resort with activities from morning 'til the "wee hours," and we were too busy making sure that our three thousand guests melted *their* tensions away to attend to our own. As the cobbler's children often went barefoot, George and I lived happily in a constant race against time.

Introduction

Worrying about twelve hundred rooms, three golf courses, forty tennis courts, three nightclubs, two pools, two health clubs, indoor and outdoor skating rinks, a ski area, plus the stars and politicians who arrived regularly, may not sound like everyone's life. But being harried isn't content-specific: in America these days, it seems that everyone is working 24/7.

Looking back, I often wonder why this illness happened to me. Did God think I needed more mountains to climb?

Many people get one cancer and learn to deal with it, but I was given two unrelated ones at the same time and didn't know it.

Misdiagnosis is a common occurrence everywhere, and my bottle of fexofenadine (Allegra), a wonder drug for allergies, remains in my medicine cabinet, a constant reminder that anyone can be given the right pills for the wrong diagnosis.

Sometimes it's difficult for doctors to come up with what's really ailing you. It can take months and regrettably even years for the real truth to emerge.

I consider myself one of the lucky ones who somehow asked the right questions early on, which led to the right answers.

Admittedly, I was afraid of cancer. I couldn't even say the word; but slowly I learned to embrace it and then squash it—kill it—stamp on it—eliminate it—with every bit of courage and strength I could muster.

Some of my friends and family are still hush-hush when it comes to speaking about cancer. But how can we help each other if we don't share information and ideas, which make cancer treatment more palatable for patients and caregivers alike?

Look Out Cancer...Here I Come! is a book about empowerment, courage, caring and ultimately making the right decisions. Every bit of advice it offers, from the patient point of view, has been reviewed and applauded by the oncologists and cancer researchers who worked so hard to save my life.

It was Dr. Goy himself who suggested that I write a book with good, easy-to-understand information and a positive attitude to help others get through their battle as well as I did. Knowing I was in the middle of another manuscript called *How To Stay Married to a Man with 1200 Bedrooms*, a light-hearted, true story of the hotel where I spent the better part of 30 years, he suggested that I put that one on the shelf for a while and concentrate on a book that would help others to get it right the first time, with sound advice from one patient to another.

Part I

The Cancer Credo

Cancer is something that crept into me...
But I can lick it; you just wait and see,
I wish I didn't have it
It's never the best.
Often I'm tired,
And just have no zest...
I have cancer, don't like it one bit—
Sometimes I cry out, "Why was I hit?"
I tried to be good, to be honest and true,
I gave of myself—it's the right thing to do.
I lived by the Good Book
Where sharing is best,
Took care of my family, and passed every test,
And yet I got it, I'll never know why.
But I'm going to beat this—*Pow* right in the eye!
I bike, and I sing, I do everything right.
I follow the program, as hard as I might...
"You can and you will,"
I say to myself,
"Let's put this cancer back up on the shelf."
Each day, when I wake up, I know what to say:
"Good-bye to you, cancer, now be on your way!"

Sharon Lee Parker

1

Follow Your Instinct!

Pretend you're happy when you're blue
It isn't very hard to do
And you'll find happiness without an end
Whenever you pretend

from "Pretend"

Sitting in the doctor's waiting room one June afternoon, I saw an elderly woman who looked so thin and pale that I had the urge to reach out and hug her. Chilly, even in summer, she was sitting alone covered in a soft warm blanket. I slid into the chair next to her and we struck up the standard conversation to be having at a cancer center.

"What kind of cancer do you have?" she asked softly.

"Hodgkin's lymphoma," I replied. "How about you?"

"I have plain old lymphoma, and it's in a late stage."

No one had to tell me that. It was evident by the sunken weariness in her eyes and the total lack of color in her face as she stared out at me from the folds of her blanket.

"You know, you're so lucky," she said. "They can cure you."

"I hope so," I said. "I'm trying so hard to do everything right."

"I am too," she said. "But I didn't find mine until it was very late. If only I had followed my instincts," she continued. In her small town in Oklahoma, her symptoms had been dismissed as the flu. Looking into her dark, sad eyes, it was clear that the mistake had been a severe one. "It's easy to want to forget you may have something serious," she continued. "It's much easier just to put it on the back burner."

"If only I had followed my instincts." The phrase seemed to echo inside me. I thought of myself, sitting next to her in my white Capris and the jaunty blue hat that my daughter Amy had made me buy.

- *My colorful way of dressing was helping to keep me upbeat, dynamic, and focused on the positive.*

The human capacity to control how reality is perceived is incredible. Something as small as a smile and a colorful hat can change your whole day. The ability to control how you perceive reality is both powerful enough to hurt you (by convincing yourself not to get that second opinion), or it can heal you through determination to believe the best, no matter what anyone says.

In my case, I was already headed to the latter group, among those lucky ones who would find the grace to triumph over cancer through determination to get well. I was going to live. I just knew it. But how did I get to that point? Looking at this white-faced, soft-spoken patient, I became aware of how frighteningly thin the line was that separated us.

"You are so lucky," she repeated, "You are truly blessed."

"So are you," I said. "I know that God is watching us both, and even though yours is tougher than mine, miracles happen every day. Let's hope that you are today's miracle."

"That's the way I live," she continued, "one day at a time."

"I know," I said, "each day we have one more mountain to climb, but we will reach the top and celebrate together."

We hugged as the receptionist called my name for the shots that would enable me to have my next "chemo cocktail."

The exchange remained imprinted in my memory for two reasons: first, the vast difference in our diagnosis seemed to be hauntingly encapsulated by her phrase, "*if I had only followed my instincts.*" Second, if events had not turned out the way they did, I could have easily been the one wearing her shoes. But a combination of factors came forward to save my life (as they may yours).

Successfully rid of two different forms of cancer, I have been on the "firing line" twice and came out on the other end perfectly healthy. But at one time I was on the brink of more serious consequences. How I managed to escape that fate—and how you can, too—is a true story of strength and determination.

Until cancer made its unwelcome visit, I could have been the lady next door, living a life of wonderful everyday happiness. I could have been your neighbor or your sister—a friendly, busy person tackling life one day at a time. Still in love with my husband after thirty-seven years of marriage, with two married children secure in their jobs and with grandchildren here and on the way, there was nothing to deny that I was living a charmed life. I had accomplished everything that was important to me, and as I approached my fifty-seventh year, I was looking forward to the new adventures that life had to offer.

But one of the cardinal rules of life is that at the moment you least expect it, everything can change. The signs were already lurking in the shadows, weeks before my diagnosis, as I left in early April to visit my daughter Amy. When I left my house, outside of Charleston, South Carolina, that morning, I was feeling a little the worse for wear. The pollen counts were quite high, and everyone in the Palmetto State seemed to be suffering from allergies. An over-the-counter allergy medication wiped the problem out of my sinuses—and out of my mind. The underlying condition would turn out to be much more difficult to alleviate, but as far as I was concerned, "no symptoms, no problem."

Convinced that cooler weather to the north was what I needed, I headed toward Washington, D.C., and checked into a hotel outside of historic McLean, Virginia, for a night's rest. A new shopping plaza had been built right across the busy thoroughfare, and forgetting that I was "under the weather," I ran over to a maternity store called Pea in the Pod and began looking for a present to take to my pregnant daughter. When a party dress caught my eye, I didn't hesitate to try it on. The store pillows I stuffed into the dress to simulate Amy's five months of pregnancy made me quite a sight; I bought it and laughed all the way to Syracuse.

During the next five days, I spent wonderful hours with my family, and even though I didn't feel quite right, I chalked it up to the long drive and exhaustion, as most people would. The suggestion that I had anything more than a common cold would have seemed laughable to me. Time flies when you're having fun, and pretty soon, I was back on the highway heading home. I felt a tiny pea-sized swelling near my collar bone which I thought was caused by a necklace adornment, but it disappeared as quickly as it came.

When I finally pulled into my driveway in historic Summerville, I felt take-your-shoes-off-and-drop exhausted. An annoying colorless phlegm had settled at the bottom of my throat, and no matter how hard I tried, I couldn't seem to cough it all up. Sound sleep was becoming impossible except when my head was elevated. I coughed like Old Faithful but didn't produce. When the cough became a real nuisance, I discussed it with my husband, George. Not having an inkling what we would soon be facing, our conversation was laid-back and easygoing: "Perhaps you should get a checkup," he suggested, "You may need an antibiotic." I agreed.

George would turn into my biggest advocate. He was always a wonderful husband, but not all wonderful husbands can keep their spirits up in times of serious duress. During the months that followed this casual morning conversation about my "cough," I came to realize the true importance of having a partner in life.

• *In order to survive the trials associated with having—and beating—cancer, everyone needs a support system. No one should have to do it alone. If you haven't been blessed with a loving family, I discuss how you can build a support system from scratch later in the book.*

At the time, the date of the doctor's appointment seemed as good as any other, but it would become etched in my memory forever, recitable as the years of wars or the names of children.

April 4, 2002

Since we were both spending the morning at the dentist's office, George offered to come along. When we arrived, the local doctor looked down my throat, listened to my chest, checked out my other vital signs, and said, "I don't think it's anything more than allergies. Look at all the pollen outside."

I glanced out the window. It was true; the cars were covered in a pale yellow dust. After all, it was "that time of year" again, and everyone else had allergies. The doctor handed me a prescription for fexofenadine (Allegra), a well-known allergy medication.

"Should I have a chest x-ray?" I heard myself asking. This didn't feel like allergies. I thought I might have bronchitis or maybe even walking pneumonia.

"I don't think its necessary," he replied. "Your chest sounds clear, but if it'll make you feel better, I'll give you authorization."

Allergies are common in my family. My dad always had phlegm and still does at ninety years of age. "Just a chip off the old block," I commented to George as we left. In my hand, I was holding the wrong diagnosis. But in my mind, I was just a stop away from the pharmacy and a clear chest.

When I got a diagnostic chest x-ray a few days later, I thought little of it. I hadn't needed an x-ray like that in many years, and other than my standard duties as a woman (one yearly trip to the gynecologist, complete with Pap test and mammogram), I hadn't had any diagnostic tests of note in recent history. Like most of us, I was checking off my yearly medical obligations and thinking it would suffice.

I always believed that I was a model of what it means to be a healthy individual, taking very good care of myself and keeping abreast of medical research. I often thought I'd be a doctor in my next life. In this one, being a loving daughter, wife, mother, and grandmother took precedence over a medical career, but I was prepared to live a long and happy life as a case study for model health; living that life as a "survival story" instead was the furthest thing from my mind.

When the doctor failed to call me with the results of my x-rays right away, I decided to call the hospital myself. When the voice on the other end of the line said, "The results show a shadow on your x-ray, and a computed tomography (CT) scan is now recommended," I was very sure I needed antibiotics and was just waiting for my appointment the next week to get an official diagnosis of walking pneumonia or bronchitis. My mind went to other projects, however, and stayed there: after I drank my morning coffee, the phlegm and my cough seemed to dissipate, and I took this clearance for the green light I needed to move on to other things.

I went alone to the hospital in Charleston. It wasn't far from our home, and besides, I thought I already knew what they were going to say. When a member of the department of radiology showed me the results of my CT scan, I couldn't believe my eyes. The bottom line declared, among other possibilities, "Suspect lymphoma or small-cell carcinoma."

"What?" I cried in a trembling voice, "This is impossible! These can't be my results...There is no history of cancer in my family. This must be a mistake!"

I was in a state of utter shock, truly believing that the hospital must have mixed up my chart with someone else's or input the wrong data into mine. After I calmed down somewhat, the radiologist gently told me that I needed to schedule an appointment with the hospital's pulmonologist as soon as possible. When I called this lung specialist's office, the young voice at the other end of the line seemed surprisingly unconcerned about my welfare. She explained to me in clear, inflexible language, that being a new patient, I would have to wait eight days for an appointment.

"I may have cancer," I wailed into the phone, "I can't wait that long! I'll come any time, day or night."

"I'm sorry, there are no exceptions," was the curt answer. "We see new patients only on certain days of the month."

If dealing with such unexpected medical results was new for me, dealing with the bureaucracy of a hospital system, in my emotional state, was even more so. I had just gotten that x-ray on a whim, and now my life was becoming unhinged because of it! The days were like a dream, and I was waiting for the moment when I'd wake up and return to my happy life. The allergy medication sat unused in my purse, now becoming a reminder of how crucial attending to your intuition can be.

George was rightly concerned and outraged when he heard how long it would take to get an appointment with the lung specialist in Charleston. He immediately called our friend Dr. Robert Press, an infectious disease specialist at NYU in New York City. Whenever serious medical problems arose in our family, Dr. Press was the one we called for sound advice.

"Fax me that report," he said calmly, "and I'll let you know what I think."

Ten minutes later, Dr. Press called back with more urgency in his voice. "I think Sharon should come to New York tomorrow," he said. "We need to find out what this thing is. Hopefully, it will turn out to be nothing serious."

In the thirty years I had known Bob Press, he had never once asked me to come to New York for medical reasons. He told me to bring my records, including the confusing CT scan of my chest. Even my newly purchased bottle of allergy medication would come along for the ride. I didn't think I had life-threatening symptoms; I didn't seem to have any of the seven cancer warning signs. What could this be? I couldn't imagine! All I knew was that I was going to New York and hoping that God was coming with me.

As I would soon realize, a silent but life-altering count-down had been going on during the trip to see my daughter—one that may have been brewing even earlier. It was marked by the "allergies" I had when I left that April afternoon, the "exhaustion" I had when I got home, and the harmless-looking "transparent phlegm" that bothered me more as a nuisance than as a harbinger of dangerous things to come. In reality, these symptoms were more dangerous than the inexplicable pain or bleeding that sends most people running to the hospital precisely because they could all be rationalized away. (I had "allergies" because of the pollen and hereditary tendencies, the "exhaustion" was from the drive, and the "phlegm" was a symptom of a viral infection or walking pneumonia at the very worst.)

- *Luckily for me, I trusted my gut instinct enough to risk annoying my doctor by asking him if I should get a chest x-ray, even though he had just finished telling me. "You have nothing more than allergies." This decision to risk seeming overly cautious and to get a chest x-ray may have saved my life.*

- *I always believed that a condition like cancer was the kind of disease that happens to somebody else—maybe even a family member or a friend but always somebody else. It isn't. It's the kind of thing that can happen to anyone, including you and me.*

My drive to find out more was what initially saved me, because unlike countless others, I didn't go home satisfied with a quick and easy explanation for the way I was feeling. My intuition told me that there was something more than allergies at work, and I listened. What made me listen? Why did I ask for that chest x-ray? Was it luck? Character? Habit? I really don't know. But I do know that I have continued to attend to my intuition and have learned to value it always.

"*If only I had followed my instincts,*" the woman in the waiting room had mused, "and become determined to go the extra mile, despite inconvenience or logic to the contrary, I might not be in this position today."

Unfortunately, there is a plethora of stories out there of people who don't survive cancer because, for whatever reason, they go home without the right diagnosis (or misdiagnose themselves without going to a doctor) and the symptoms of cancer are explained away all too easily...only to resurface later, worse and nastier, ready to wipe out the entire person.

Sometimes a patient observes the symptoms, goes to the doctor, gets a misdiagnosis, and receives a medication that relieves the symptoms, only to find out weeks, months, or even years later that cancer has shown up "out of nowhere." I know this can happen because it almost happened to me.

- *The determination to take an extra proactive step is what uncovered my cancer, but it is also what ultimately healed me. If you're holding this book, you probably know that a day like any other can turn into a day of destiny, changing your life forever. But even if the diagnosis is cancer, those changes don't have to be for the worse.*

This is a story about love, determination, and what it takes to survive and triumph. When the doctors told me I had cancer, I didn't crumple into a heap and stay there. I did my best to face my foe bravely, and say "*Look Out Cancer...Here I Come!*" And you know what? I'm here today to tell you that it worked. When you're finished reading this book and going through your treatments, you won't be *wishing* you had followed your instincts. You'll be thanking God that you attended to every thought they had to offer.

2

The Road to Realization

Whenever I feel afraid
I hold my head erect
And whistle a happy tune
So no one will suspect I'm afraid…

from "Whistle a Happy Tune"

Leaving Charleston, South Carolina, I was clinging to an overnight bag as if squeezing it could somehow allay my anxiety. It was already not an easy trip, and I hadn't even left the platform to board the train to New York.

George had offered to come along, but with my typical "I'm fine, I can do it" attitude, I reassured him that it wasn't necessary, and he left on a business trip. Not wholly un-aware that I might need some assistance, my dear friend Evelyn had come with me to offer her support, and I knew that I would find some encouragement in her dancing blue eyes and upbeat attitude. But perhaps not enough. With one hand clutching Evelyn and the other in a white-knuckled grip on my overnight bag, I was in the prediagnostic twilight zone, barely suitable for travel.

Tears seemed to wait for me, an omnipresent force just below the surface. I felt them threatening to erupt even as I purchased my train ticket. The station attendant was a very friendly southern gentleman, and when I said, "I'll take an overnight sleeper to New York," my voice sounded perfectly calm and under control. But when he replied, "I'm sorry. All of our sleeping space has been reserved," that thin barrier of control was upset. I burst into tears, and while they streamed

17

down my face, I told him, "Fine, I'll take whatever you have." He must have figured I was in emotional turmoil (or a true sleeper-car enthusiast). But bursting into tears at unexpected intervals is a natural response to high levels of fear and anxiety, so it's important to be aware of the heightened sensitivities of a cancer patient.

* *A real cancer scare can make anyone—and I mean anyone—grab for a Kleenex and ask "Why me."*

I had always believed myself to be a strong woman (and had proven it by helping to run our renowned family business, the Concord Hotel, in upstate New York for years, raising two children, and performing a wide variety of impossible feats that I won't enumerate here). Nonetheless, despite all my composure and fifty-something years of self-control, I could be reduced to tears by the simple phrase "suspect lymphoma or small-cell carcinoma."

* *The level of vulnerability that cancer or the fear of cancer brings out is amazing. Therefore anyone dealing with cancer patients or nearly anyone dealing with a frightening diagnosis, should be aware of this sensitivity.*

Like most prediagnostic patients, I swung between two states: the suspicion that I might have cancer threw me into a state of despair, while the thought that it was something less serious would tempt me to forget the whole thing. But then, the thought that I might actually have cancer would begin the cycle of despair and denial all over again. What would happen when I got to New York? Were those serious irregularities on my CT scan? Where was all this going? Then: Were will I have dinner tonight? What will I wear tomorrow?

Patients may not be the logical, self-possessed characters you have always known. Behind the curtains, they are dancing in a strange circle between relative normalcy and total anguish. Fear can bring out all sorts of things in people, and you never know what it might bring up next.

For me, it was mainly tears. But for others, it could be anger, resentment or even regret.

• *If you're living or working with a cancer patient, the important thing is not to judge them when they display these emotions. If you are a cancer patient, the same rule applies: hold off on judging yourself when a trial like this elicits some irrationality. It inevitably will.*

• *If you are assisting with cancer patients, there is an upside to all this: the intense vulnerabilities and sensitivities etch your kindness in stone. When you interact with a patient, your kindness and care will never be forgotten.*

Frequently, we miss opportunities to do nice things for people because we feel that our efforts won't be appreciated or recognized. Perhaps others have been ungrateful to us in the past or overlooked our good deeds. But the slightest smile or indication of empathy can move a cancer patient instantly from despair and fear to hope. If there was ever a time to give of yourself, this is it. People may not react with gratitude at the moment, but don't be dissuaded. They will remember.

For instance, I have never forgotten how the stationmaster finally procured a sleeper for me to New York, or how Evelyn followed me up I-95 to make sure I would be okay. Acts that would normally grow dim with the passing years remain vivid and filled with appreciation. My feeling of gratitude also does not ebb. If you know a cancer patient, your attention and energy will never be lost.

When it came time for me to leave Evelyn and the stationmaster, I climbed aboard with the knowledge that I was leaving my friend behind greatly concerned for my well-being. Luckily, I slept all the way to New York.

April 15, 2002

When I arrived in the city, my night's rest had refreshed me, and the Big Apple seemed to have a stimulating effect, with bright sunlight pouring over all the taxicabs and hurried New Yorkers rushing along to a million different places. The first appointment I had was with the gynecologist I had trusted for more than twenty years, Dr. Charles Debrovner.

Dr. Debrovner was the kind of doctor associated with a time before HMOs: a stable and steady figure in our lives for more than two decades, he was always full of wisdom and sound advice. He was among the top in his class at Yale, and I valued his opinion greatly. Like everyone, in emergencies we rely on those we trust the most.

"Whatever you have, it will be fixable," Dr. Debrovner said confidently, once I had been seated in his office. If something were wrong with my health, he assured me, Dr. Francis Adams, a well-respected pulmonologist, would get to the bottom of it. Dr. Adams was my next appointment of the day. I thanked Dr. Debrovner for his encouragement and fairly bounced out of the office.

The blue sky outdoors brought a surge of optimism in me. With a new spring in my step, I headed toward Dr. Adams' office with budding confidence. Cancer was beginning to sound more like a bad dream than a condition actually inside my body.

When I arrived at Dr. Adams' office, he was very genial, and he remembered my visit to him with bronchitis years ago; this bolstered my faith in him. This wasn't the harried doctor you sometimes see on daytime TV—those who are overly rushed and forced to cut corners. This was the best kind of doctor you could get—caring, careful, skillful, and highly respected. He didn't seem overly worried about my case either, but he nonetheless wanted to test me. A technician came in and set up a machine into which I had to breathe and then hold my breath. "Breathe!" the technician said at least a hundred times. But Dr. Adams said my lungs seemed quite normal, so all the huffing and puffing was worth the effort.

"I think this may be a sarcoid or granulomatous disease, both of which we can successfully treat."

Relieved, I felt that life had just been infused back to me. "Sometimes these diseases even go away by themselves," he continued, "but we need to be certain. Given the results of your CT scans, I want you to go and see Dr. Bernie Crawford."

"Who is he?" I asked, fearing more marathon tests.

"He's the man who will evaluate everything we've done today, and he'll decide whether a biopsy is in order. We want to make sure you're treated for the right condition."

It all sounded reasonable and safe. I took his advice, and scheduled an appointment with Dr. Crawford for the following day. Each visit to a doctor was boosting my self-assurance a little more, inflating my confidence slowly like a colorful balloon that I couldn't wait to tie off and put in the air. I was going to be fine!

On the way back, I stopped to see Bob Press at the NYU Medical Center to thank him for his help. "What do you think?" I asked him, feeling better every second. "Your blood work is perfectly normal," he reasoned aloud, "except for the sedimentation rate, which was slightly elevated. Let's see what Bernie has to say. He's our 'guru' in cases like these." So this was it: after my many meetings, there was one more expert to see who would, hopefully, confirm the good news.

The next day, I was ready to get things wrapped up at this "guru's" office and turn a somber visit into a real vacation. Optimism is contagious, and my three doctors so far were all helpful. George had arrived from Florida: he was planning to come with me to Dr. Crawford's office, and then we would go together to our favorite Italian restaurant, Patsy's, on West 56th Street, which would be a comfort after bad news and a great place to celebrate good news.

As I got ready for my appointment with Dr. Crawford the next day, I decided to go ahead and dress for our evening out. To tell the truth, I wasn't feeling chipper, but I wanted so much to be told I was well that, subconsciously, I

21

wanted to prove to Dr. Bernie Crawford, with my outfit and demeanor, that I was healthy. After all, how could you tell someone in a cute silk dress and high heels, wearing lipstick and looking ten years younger than she ought, that she had cancer? It wasn't logical, but as I said, fear brings out the un-expected.

- *A psychologist might have told me I was in "denial." But paradoxically, as you will see throughout my story, it was precisely this denial—the refusal to believe the worst, the determination to keep fighting for the best, the high-spir-ited denial of sinking despair that would ultimately help me.*

April 17, 2002

Dr. Crawford was a thoroughly esteemed and experi-enced surgeon at the NYU Medical Center. He had an edu-cated, highly professional air and immediately made me feel more at ease. "You were probably rushed here," he told me as he gestured for us to sit down. He didn't seem worried or anxious, even though he had clearly read my file, and per-haps didn't want to frighten me unnecessarily.

"What about my CT scan?" I asked him.

"I'm not sure what caused this unexpected result," he answered.

"What do you recommend?" George asked seriously.

"Well, we could do a biopsy, or we could watch it and wait a bit," he replied. I had already considered the latter op-tion. Even my concerned sister Ellen was advocating a "wait-and-see-attitude" and had sent me a computer printout of sarcoid diseases.

"What would you do if I were your wife?" I interjected, hoping he would say, "I'd do nothing now," and we could get on to Patsy's, where I knew a big plate of veal Parmesan and a friendly environment were waiting for me.

He pondered the question for a moment.

"If you were my wife, I would biopsy a lymph node at the base of your neck, just to make sure it wasn't serious." My pulse quickened at the thought. "I'm convinced," he continued, "there's a 65 percent chance this is sarcoidosis and a 30 percent chance it's granulomas. Both are very treatable disorders. There remains, however, a 5 percent probability that this is a form of lymphoma."

"Lymphoma…" the word flew in my right ear and out the left. I knew nothing about lymphoma and didn't want to know more. Who cares about a 5 percent chance of anything? Ninety-five percent odds were good enough for me.

At this point, my path was already riddled with opportunities to give up the hot pursuit of this elusive enigma and get back to my normal life. I could have just waited the eight days for the visit in Charleston. I could have convinced myself that it was hopefully nothing serious from my three highly respected doctors and gone home to "wait and see," could have…

But George was adamant: "As long as we're here, you should have the procedure and get to the bottom of this."

There was no use arguing with his logic, even though I felt ready to pack up my bags and head home. Once again, it was a high level of determination (this time George's, not mine) that would lead to a key discovery. My determination had made the x-ray happen; George's was bringing the biopsy into being. The frightening thing in all this is how easily those things could have been disregarded. I didn't have to ask Dr. Crawford what he would have done if I were his wife. George didn't have to suddenly become adamant that I get the biopsy. The opportunities to go home—and unwittingly walk into cancer's trap—abounded. But this highly skilled surgeon assured me it would be a simple snip of a tiny tissue and that it would help them establish the indicated treatment as soon as possible. I got all the persuasion I needed. But how many people don't? How many people go home to wait and see, because its less threatening, and wind up seeing something they never intended to be a part of their lives?

Walking out of that doctor's office, I felt very good. I had now seen four highly respected doctors in two days, and although they were concerned, none was overly alarmed by my case. The biopsy was a just-in-case measure. The 5 percent chance that it would show something serious floated away with the passing of the hours. Maybe this would turn into a pleasure trip, after all...

At Patsy's, George and I had a warm and intimate dinner nestled in the familiar chairs along the wall. Frank Sinatra had been a longtime patron, and it was fun to reminisce about all the famous people that had passed in and out of Patsy's doors. As we sat there together talking and laughing, George and I were optimistic. A chorus of doctors was giving me no cause for panic, and if we were that lucky, great. Otherwise, we would beat it, whatever it was. As we left the restaurant, I slipped my hand into George's and felt the special kind of warmth and caring that grows especially strong in a good marriage. I knew I was going to be fine because I was in good hands, both the trusted hands of my doctors and the loving hands of George.

We both decided to go to a Broadway play after dinner. That was what tourists did in New York, right? That city is a bustling town and a great place to forget things. We walked all the way to the box office, and with each step I took, my spirits seemed to rise, until it was all yesterday's news. Did I have a deep uncertainty in the back of my mind? Yes. Was I intent on smothering it, crushing it, and totally obliterating it? Yes. I pounded it into the pavement with every step, crowded it out with positive thinking, and chased it off further with every laugh. A musical, *The Producers*, was showing. It was a comedy, and laughter was right up my alley. There were two tickets left. I was thrilled. We were in New York; I was going to be fine! There's nothing like a comedy to make you forget your troubles. We discussed the amusing points of the show and laughed all the way back to the hotel. It would be the last time we did so for a very long time.

3

It's Impossible

It's impossible
Tell the sun to leave the sky
It's just impossible...
Ask a baby not to cry
It's just impossible...

from "It's Impossible"

April 18, 2002

The next day found me on the sixth floor of NYU Medical Center's Rusk Institute for outpatient surgery. In the examining room, I changed into hospital garb and tried to stay calm by singing to myself. Dr. Crawford had brought up a biopsy only after I had asked him what he would do if I were his wife. To my way of thinking, that meant it was probably just a security measure, right?

A nurse came by to ask me about my allergies and other historical information, followed by the anesthesiologist. He was good-looking, young, and friendly, and I felt that I recognized him from somewhere. "You look so familiar," I said, "Just like a Concord Hotel guest." He looked at me quizzically. "Our family used to be the owners," I explained.

"Well, to tell the truth, my Aunt Gladys married a member of your family, and I was a guest at your hotel many times," he replied, somewhat dumbfounded.

"We're all connected," I piped in happily. Now I was beginning to feel better. I wasn't an anonymous patient being snipped in Outpatient Surgery—a family member, albeit a distant one, would be looking out for me in the operating room.

We chatted about fond memories for a few moments, and then we got down to business. "Why are you here?" he asked me.

"To rule out lymphoma," I replied matter-of-factly. Soon, he was putting a mask gently over my nose and mouth.

"Count to ten Sharon, you'll be just fine... One... two... three..."

I awoke in a large, crowded recovery room. It was obvious that my biopsy was not the only surgery for the day. My throat felt parched and dry, and when a nurse approached and asked me how I was feeling, I asked her if I could have some water. The answer was no. "But I'll get you an ice chip," she added quickly.

My mouth felt as if I had spent the morning crawling across the Sahara, and the ice chip was ridiculously wonderful against my scorched throat. A few moments later, I moved my hand up my neck, feeling a bandage right under my voice box but none on my chest. That made me think. The doctor had mentioned that he would stop the biopsy as soon as he could get a definite diagnosis. It looked like he must have found something. But what? I was trying to remain positive, but a feeling of uncertainty suddenly swept over me.

I didn't have to wonder for long. A few minutes later, Dr. Crawford stopped by the recovery room. "I am really surprised and sorry," he said, looking me squarely in the eye. "Classic Hodgkin's lymphoma is the preliminary diagnosis. It's treatable. Now, get some rest."

I didn't cry. I was too stunned to cry. How could this be? I could deal with walking pneumonia or sarcoidosis; but Hodgkin's lymphoma. What *was* Hodgkin's lymphoma, anyway? That meant cancer, the "Big C." But for me, the "Big C" stood for the Concord, not for cancer! I didn't even want to think about it. "This can't be happening to me," I thought as I again drifted off to sleep.

It's Impossible

It would have sounded absurd to me at the time, but in truth I had a lot to be thankful for, lying on that hospital bed in the NYU Medical Center recovery room. First, I had listened to my intuition and gone past the initial allergy misdiagnosis. Second, I had taken George's advice and pursued the biopsy even though it hadn't been presented as a "must" at the time. These two factors combined made a complete recovery possible; whereas if I had gone back home to "wait and see," I very well might have waited too long and seen something too terrible to imagine for my whole family. From a bird's-eye perspective, knowing what I know now, that decision to have a biopsy played a vital role in saving my life and was one of the best decisions I've ever made. But at the time, the results made it seem like the worst day of my life, and it would take a while for my perceptions to change.

As I awoke again, I remembered that I had just been told there was lymphoma swimming around in my chest.

"Why me?" I whispered to myself. I wondered how many other people in the recovery room had the same question on their minds. Were there others, like me, lying only a few hospital beds away? Or was I the only one, the winner of the bad-news lottery for the day?

Did God really think I needed another mountain to climb? I didn't even know what Hodgkin's lymphoma was, much less how I got it. All I knew was that cancer cells were multiplying somewhere in my body.

When I was released from the surgical unit, George came in and helped me into a cab. We were headed toward the Marriott on 53rd Street, where I could heal from the minor surgery and await further instructions. I had to face it: I had Hodgkin's disease, whatever that was. George was in denial.

"It's impossible," he'd say, "you only have little ailments, never anything major."

He called my ninety-year-old dad to give him the news because it was hard for me to speak. Disbelieving, and always skeptical of doctors, Dad just said, "Tell her I love her."

I knew my mom, Cecilia, must be very confused, worried, and wondering where I was because I usually stopped by my parents' condominium in Palm Beach for leisurely walks with our two English setters, McCoy and McKenzie. When I later told her I had cancer, she cried but only remembered it for a few minutes. She was eighty-seven and suffering from short-term memory loss. She was full of wisdom and advice, but her mind was cloudy about the present. Now it would be up to my sister Ellen to take more of the load of family responsibilities.

Self-pity aside (and if I had chosen to, I could have drowned in that), there was a ton of planning to do. Cancer was an uninvited and very demanding guest. I still couldn't believe I had it. No one in my family had cancer. "Doesn't run in the genes," my dad would proudly quip whenever the subject of disease came up. But regardless of whether or not it *seemed* real to me, my focus would have to be on how, when, and where to lick this thing quickly and permanently. Crumpling up into a ball and hoping it would all go away was not an option. Maybe I couldn't talk because my throat was still sore from the surgery, but I could plan.

What would I tell the children and the rest of the family? What about George? How would my husband handle all this in the long term? Did I need a second opinion, or even a third? Would the medical centers near home be the best equipped to treat me? Alternatively, would I have to move somewhere? For how long? How were our dogs, locked up in a kennel in Summerville, South Carolina, faring? I started to cry, and as the cries turned to sobs, they hurt the incision below my neck. In whom could I confide? Who were the people to trust? My mind was reeling. The trip from allergies to cancer had been a short one, and I was still dizzy from the descent.

Suddenly, I heard myself saying sternly, "Get a grip, Sharon! You are strong! You can beat this monster!" I didn't know where it was coming from, but a rising tide of confidence and determination was welling up inside me. And I knew that if I kept it flowing, my chances of beating cancer would be at their best.

4

The Search for the Cure!

When you walk through a storm
Hold your head up high...
And don't be afraid of the dark.
At the end of the storm
There's a golden sky...
from "You'll Never Walk Alone"

April 20, 2002

A very light tap on my shoulder startled me out of a deep sleep. As I opened my eyes, standing in front of me was our son John who'd flown in from Houston, Texas, to New York. "You are a delight for sore eyes," I whispered to him. "What time is it?"

"It's 10 P.M. I'm sorry. My plane was late."

I was thrilled to see him again. His deep-set brown eyes and infectious smile always put me in a good mood. He gave me a loving hug and sat down beside me.

- *Coming to the "rescue" in a timely fashion can have a positive impact on the psyche of one who has been diagnosed with cancer. It shows the patient that he or she is not alone and eases this new burden.*

John had demonstrated good sound judgment and had proven many times in the past that he was wise beyond his years. As a general manager for Marriott International, he'd become a decision maker. Growing up in a hotel setting and working from the time he was a young boy hadn't hurt him one bit.

He leaned over and kissed me on the cheek. "You'll be fine mom, whatever this is, we'll beat it." How I loved hearing those words. He sounded so convincing, and I knew that George deeply appreciated having such positive support arrive so quickly. Amy, now in her sixth month of pregnancy, would be landing at LaGuardia the following morning.

- *The diagnosis of any serious illness is traumatic for everyone involved. Having a support system is key to holding it all together.*

After thirty-seven years of marriage, we would face our toughest test all together as a family, because of a tiny piece of tissue removed from below my neck and placed under a microscope. I wondered how the doctors could see so much and be so positive about the preliminary diagnosis. It was all happening too fast. Talking was impossible. The many questions and concerns that whirled through my mind would have to wait.

- *In a time of emotional and physical stress, it's always smart to listen to the ideas of others whom you trust.*

George brought me a large pad and a red pen saying in the gentlest of ways, "Don't speak now. Write everything down and save your voice." I looked into his tired sad eyes and knew that he was crying inside, but he never let me see the tears. He was a loving, caring person and perhaps, the finest man I'd ever known. The ups and downs of marriage had forged strong bonds between us. Adding to the burdens of his life was the last thing I ever wanted to do.

Feeling unsure about the next step to take, I simply wrote, "Thank you," wanting everyone to know how much I appreciated their support. George had been through plenty of turmoil in his life, yet he was blessed with an indomitable spirit and always looked to the future. He simply didn't let life's problems get him down; I remembered that quality and decided that I should try to react in the same proactive way.

John had the same optimism. He was positive from day one and could usually fix a problem or straighten out a situation before it grew into something major. Could I catch that quality from him? *"Think positive,"* a little voice whispered from within.

"I want you to consider M.D. Anderson, Houston," I suddenly heard my son say. "It's rated the top cancer hospital in the country, and we'll be there with you every step of the way."

- *We'll be there with you every step of the way." The importance of that phrase can't be overstated. It shows support, commitment, and strength to cancer patients and reminds them that they are not alone.*

As John kissed me goodnight, ever so gently, my eyes welled up with tears. Perhaps, he was on the right track by suggesting that George and I move to Texas to be treated at a renowned cancer center; but at the time, it sounded monumental and more than I wanted to consider.

John had an uncanny ability to tell when something wasn't going well just by the tone of a person's voice. His idea bounced back and forth as I tried to fall back asleep.

It would be reassuring to be near him and my daughter-in-law Chrissy. Now that I was aware that Houston was a leader in cancer research, it gave me a lot to ponder as I wrestled with this new idea. Still, I was in New York City, and NYU Medical Center had diagnosed me without delay. Memorial Sloan-Kettering was also a leader in cancer research. I'd have to get more opinions and suggestions before making any final decisions. At least my brain had plenty to work with as I floated into a deeper sleep; but one idea kept repeating itself: "Get it right the first time."

Early the next morning, Amy arrived with love in her heart and tears in her eyes. She was very pregnant once again, but as a mother, I thought she was the most beautiful "lady in waiting" I'd ever seen. A heightened realization that your days have a cloud hanging over them makes any pleasure that you receive even greater.

Our daughter was a goal setter and would offer sound advice and good judgment. We must have done something right, I thought, as I listened carefully to her words of wisdom. "Don't make any hasty decisions that you may regret. Look at all of your options and decide where you'll be the most comfortable. You always need a second opinion in instances like this. As long as you're in New York, let's make some calls."

Following her sage advice, we agreed on a plan. Two oncologists in New York, Dr. Kenneth Hymes at NYU Medical Center and Dr. Andrew Zelenetz at Memorial Sloan-Kettering, were the choices.

- *Having your family together gives you tremendous support and direction, something everyone needs at a time like this. Not only has your immune system been compromised, but your emotional system and ability to make wise decisions are impaired as well. Listening to the ideas of those who really love you will help you get through this nightmare.*

It was decided that I would accept an invitation to spend a week with our beloved friends Evelyn and Charles Cathcart in Tuxedo Park, New York, while undergoing more examinations and tests. They were part of our family in the truest sense and had been there from the onset. All of us felt a bond with them, which had been cemented long before, and it would be a "tonic" to go back to Tuxedo, where we had loved life for more than twenty years. The Cathcarts invited us to stay in their historic home; we looked forward to grabbing a bit of the past and clinging to it for old times' sake.

- *Every cancer patient wants to go back to the way things were, but that never lasts for long. We need to move forward and look hopefully to the future.*

"The clean mountain air of Tuxedo Park will do you good," Evelyn had urged convincingly. "I'll be happy to drive you back into the city for any appointments you need."

- *Friends can make a big difference in the way you cope. Evelyn loved me no matter what. For those sharing cancer experiences this is a very important message to convey.*

Now I was praying that I really had Hodgkin's disease instead of non-Hodgkin's lymphoma, because Dr. Crawford had mentioned to George that "it's easier to cure." What a difference a few days can make. Naturally, I was hoping that he had made a huge error, that the wrong slides were analyzed, that my name was mixed up with someone else's. I didn't want to be sick. I wanted my body to thrive. Dozing off with that thought in mind, I dreamed that I had an infection. "Take some penicillin; get some rest; in a few days you'll be as good as new." In the morning, George would make me coffee and then go off to work, where he'd convince the world that steel structures for the home were the construction solution for the twenty-first century. By now, George had retired from the hotel business and had taken over management of a company that sold light-gauge steel for residential and commercial properties.

The telephone rang in the hotel room, jolting me out of this blissful dream. I didn't answer it; I just let it ring and ring. At that moment I didn't want to admit to anyone else that I'd let myself get sick with cancer—that most insidious disease. Could it be that I'd set the groundwork by not taking care of myself? Indeed, I'd forgotten about resting, relaxing and trying to reduce the overwhelming stress that invaded my life from time to time. Could that have been the trigger? I wasn't sure, but I definitely wanted to find out. Whatever the cause, I knew that I would soon pay a dear price.

5

Putting the Pieces Together

Climb ev'ry mountain,
Search high and low
Follow ev'ry by-way,
Every path you know
from "Climb Every Mountain"

Recalling the events of 9/11 sent chills through my body. My mind often darted back to that fateful day on I-95, heading south, when I heard the news that a plane had hit the World Trade Center. It was nearly 9 A.M., and I'd already driven four hours on my weekly commute from Summerville, South Carolina, to Boca Raton, Florida, for a check on our house and a mandatory visit with Mom and Dad.

"How tragic, and how scary for the people inside the building," I heard myself say, as I neared St. Augustine. "Another plane has just hit the World Trade Center." Listening to the radio announcer, unable to digest what he was saying, I quickly called George who was already hard at work in Summerville.

"Have you heard what's going on in New York?" I asked.

"I can't believe it," he replied, incredulously.

I kept driving, listening, and praying silently for the people. It was hard to fathom that terrorists were attacking our country, just as it would become difficult to accept the fact that something was attacking me from within. Later that week, we learned the dismal truth: that thousands of people were dead. For months I couldn't pull myself away from CNBC, CNN, or Fox News.

Now, seven months later, I had a terrorist inside my body, but I was on the ground and was determined to fight back. I remembered those who weren't so lucky and felt very grateful for the chance to attack this foreign invader.

Knowing that I needed to get those second opinions, I headed back to NYU Medical Center to Kenneth Hymes, a hematologist/oncologist. As I entered his waiting room dressed as if I were going to a matinee, I still found it hard to admit anything to anyone, including myself. The room was crowded with people who looked pale and sad. "Could all of these people have cancer?" I mumbled to myself, wanting to leave right then.

Slowly, I ventured up to the receptionist, longing for a friendly face, but being preoccupied, she didn't seem to notice me. I sat back down. My name was called an hour later. Reality set in as I was escorted to an examining room and told to remove my clothes and put on a hospital gown. I didn't want to be a cancer patient; I wanted to be that receptionist.

Dr. Hymes listened attentively to my story and had the final report of the biopsy faxed over to him. "Let's do a bone marrow test and see if this cancer has spread," this sage oncologist suggested.

I agreed, having no idea what I was in for. As I sat there on the table, I asked him the question that I would repeat over and over again for the next year to anyone who would listen: "What did I do wrong?"

"You did nothing wrong," he replied gently. "It just happened. We don't have all the answers as to why or who comes down with it. Perhaps we'll know in the future."

"Can I be cured?" It's a question that looms large on a cancer patient's mind.

"That depends on how far it has traveled," he replied. "Hodgkin's is a contiguous disease. It spreads from node to node." Not knowing if I was doomed, I sat alone as the doctor left the cool room, preparing for the bone marrow test. I felt chilled and in a daze as reality set in. I had cancer; now, I'd be lucky to be a survivor. He soon returned and a large needle went into my lower back. I hollered, probably louder than necessary. It really hurt, and I wondered how many patients I scared out of the waiting room. Like many newly diagnosed patients, I was feeling sorry for myself.

I'd already been pinched, x-rayed, scanned, bruised, and biopsied in a very short time. There was a scar on my neck right under the Adam's apple to prove it. Now, my hip bone had another scar, made for the sake of gathering more data.

- *Information can save your life. The more you have, the better the chance for the best treatment.*

It didn't take long for Dr. Hymes to read the report. The bone marrow was not involved. I was so relieved. This negative report was a sign that the cancer had not spread into other regions of my body. Maybe I could be cured after all. I thanked Dr. Hymes profusely for giving me the first ray of hope and left with a smile, albeit a little one, on my face.

- *Celebrating every good piece of news is a priority for every cancer patient.*

The next morning it was time to meet Dr. Andrew Zelenetz, Chief of Lymphoma Services, Sloan-Kettering for his words of advice. A whole new world of cancer opened up before my eyes, which I had a hard time accepting. There were so many people in the lobby. The receptionist gave me a number and told me to take the elevator to the fourth floor. I sat down in the waiting room once again, but this time for no clear reason I lost my composure and began to sob.

A lovely lady came from behind the desk and gave me a hug. Her name was Erin and she had seen this happen many times before. Eventually I met Dr. Andrew Zelenetz, who was a tall, imposing figure. He had a fine reputation in the lymphoma world and I knew that I was lucky to be seeing him. I was hoping for a kind doctor who would tell me, "You'll be fine." No one was saying that just yet...

He tried to make me feel better by sharing the fact that he had treated my father-in-law, Ray Parker, for late-stage lymphoma. "It was more serious than yours," he offered, hoping to lift my spirits. It didn't work. I wasn't ready to accept it.

I remember the diagnosis well, and wondered if cancer is contagious. He soon redirected the conversation back to why I was in his office.

"I want you to get an echocardiogram of your heart and a CT scan of your chest, abdomen, and pelvis. We want to be sure that this hasn't spread," the doctor urged.

I'd already had a positron emission tomography (PET) scan, a bone marrow biopsy, twenty-four tubes of blood taken, a lymph node biopsy, and answered a pot full of questions. "How much more testing will be needed?" I asked, hoping I'd soon be done.

"This is just the beginning," he said gently. "You are in for quite a siege." I didn't want to believe it. All I wanted was my life back the way it used to be. We said our farewells after I had promised that I would listen to him and go through every necessary diagnostic test that he required.

As I drove through the hectic New York traffic back to bucolic Tuxedo Park, Evelyn was at my side. I thought to myself how fortunate I was to be seen by such reputable doctors.

"I'm in big trouble," I said to her, explaining how many tests I still needed before any treatment could be entertained.

"But you're also a fighter. You can beat this," she said in her upbeat way.

I started to repeat over and over again: *"I can beat this... I can beat this... I can beat this...."*

- *You will learn to love that phrase. You just have to say it often enough and begin to believe it.*

The following day I fasted for the scans, the first of many that would be performed at the East River Imaging Center, in New York. Feeling a bit more in control of my life, I decided to call my dear friend Manda Sanandaji, who also lived in Tuxedo Park. Her husband, Mehrdad, was a well-known internist and hematologist in neighboring Ridgewood, New Jersey.

- *Seeking out friends is a healthy way to get that extra ounce of comfort cancer patients need.*

The news had trickled down in the small village and Manda insisted on picking me up at Evelyn's house so that her husband could talk to me privately in their living room that evening. He was so gentle and concerned. After I had shown him my test results, he wrote down his best advice and talked to me about taking vitamins, also reminding me to mention *Helicobacter pylori* to the oncologist. This was a bacterium that had attacked the lining of my stomach wall some ten years before. I will never forget his kindness and concern for my well-being.

- *People who offer their hands, hearts, and brains to us in times of uncertainty give us the greatest gifts that we, as patients, can receive.*

What perhaps intrigued me the most about being stricken with cancer was that I, like many others, was used to being a giver, not a receiver. I wasn't sure how to accept all this love and attention and had to come to the realization that caring for each other is give and take. Did I think I didn't deserve it? I didn't know the answer.

- *All cancer patients are entitled to receive all the love and concern that comes their way. It's a necessary ingredient in the plan for the cure.*

The following week, I spent most of my time undergoing every conceivable test that might show how far my cancer had spread. East River Imaging proved to be a very pleasant experience after all, considering the reason I was there. I had to fast and then drink chalky-tasting barium, but the music was soothing and the surroundings were beautiful. I knew it was going to take a lot of pretending just to retain my sanity.

I wasn't going through $12,000 worth of scans. I was visiting an elegant spa! I wasn't sipping barium. It was a "banana daiquiri!"

- *It's amazing what your subconscious mind can fool your conscious brain into believing! Try it. It really works.*

All the test results were finally sent back to Dr. Zelenetz at Memorial Sloan-Kettering and I paid him another visit, more confident than before. I had done everything he had asked. Would I be out of the woods now?

"Consider yourself a very lucky young lady," he said genially, as I walked into his office a few days later. "Hodgkin's, stage IIA, is definitely what you have. This we can cure, but you're going to have to do it the old-fashioned way."

"What exactly do you mean?" I asked, feeling a bit unsure of what was coming next.

"What I mean is six months of chemotherapy and perhaps radiation." I was speechless for a change. It was more than I wanted to absorb, and perhaps he saw the reaction on my face.

"Not every week," he quickly added; "every other week."

Confused, tired, but somehow determined, I took notes as he spoke.

- *Writing down the doctor's advice is very important for future reference.*

"Where is your immediate family?" he continued.

"Syracuse, Houston, and South Carolina," I answered, without knowing where this was leading.

"Sharon, I have to be perfectly frank: You can't do this alone, and you need to be near family. You'll need all their support and to be near a major hospital."

This was all so surprising. I felt completely uneducated about chemotherapy and woefully unprepared to accept everything being thrown my way. My world was turned upside down, but I knew deep in my heart I was in some way blessed by having only Hodgkin's disease. I wasn't sure what to say.

"Perhaps, I could visit my friends and relatives in the New York area, without staying too long in any one place?" I asked hopefully.

He smiled at me. "Sharon, at your age, this is potentially serious, and you will be at risk of infection once you start treatment. You need to be nearby so you can be closely monitored."

- *Wherever you live, try to be in one place as close to a hospital as you can. If you are not living near the hospital where you are being treated, make sure the local hospital has access to your records in case of an emergency.*

Again my mind was reeling! I started to think about my husband and my life in Florida. He needed to be in the South, where steel was being used in residential construction. The dogs were another matter; I wanted them with me. I didn't want to scatter us and break up our little family. The New York rents had skyrocketed. Suddenly, I remembered

41

what my Grandma Pauline, up in Danby, Vermont, used to say: "Remember that the best is never too good."

I knew from deep within me that whatever sacrifices it took, I needed to give this my best shot. Instantly the answer became very clear: I would fly to Houston, to the M.D. Anderson Cancer Center, as John had so aptly suggested. We would make a plan. George could drive the dogs out west. Perhaps, Houstonians would be open to learning about the benefits of steel structures, in the face of termites, tornadoes, and hurricanes.

Dr. Andrew Zelenetz highly touted Dr. André Goy, a colleague who had trained at Sloan-Kettering and was on its faculty, but was now at another world-class hospital in Houston.

I could see the relief on my husband's face when we discussed the decision.

- *All cancer families need to pick a direction and go for it.*

Saying good-bye to our dear friends Evelyn and Charles wouldn't be easy. I knew they would be on the East Coast, but the best all-around plan for me was to head west. I thought of Horace Greeley and started to smile while sipping green tea in Evelyn's kitchen. "Go West young man and grow with the country!"

George and I had lived in Boulder, Colorado, years before, where I had directed a large volunteer program for seniors while teaching gerontology at the University of Northern Colorado in Greeley. Those were such good times. Perhaps we would now have some more of them. We loved the West and decided to look at it as our next adventure in life. My children had suggested that I live with them during treatment, but Amy and John both agreed that this was the right move.

- *Treatment is a chance for a new beginning and is not the end.*

- *Cancer patients need to be on a mission. Say good-bye to cancer and hello to the rest of your life.*

Before I could blink, John sent a Continental Airlines "e-ticket" to the Newark Airport Marriott, where I'd spend my last night in the New York area. Later I found out that he mentioned to the airline reservationist that I was a new M.D. Anderson cancer patient. George was already driving south to pick up the dogs, as well as his computers so he could work out of Houston, which made me feel better. Everyone knew that it would be a fight for life and that we needed to go.

6

Go West Young Woman

Though April showers may come your way,
They bring the flowers that bloom in May,
So if it's raining, have no regrets,
Because it isn't raining rain you know,
It's raining violets...

from "April Showers"

April 28, 2002

On a rainy April day, as the storm clouds gathered, I flew from New York to Houston. I sat alone in the early hours of the morning, waiting to board my plane, still holding onto the same overnight bag I had when I boarded the train in Charleston. I was traveling far from home because we were all convinced, M.D. Anderson in Houston would give me my best chance. Like everything in life, this was a gamble, but the stakes were high. For that reason we were uprooting our lives looking for the most experienced doctor in the best location for us.

As I sat waiting in the Newark airport terminal, a hard rain came pouring down. The sky lit up from lightning strikes. I had never been a great flier, but somehow none of that bothered me now. All I wanted was to be well again, and if God was leading me to M.D. Anderson—so be it. I knew I needed to have faith. I got up and walked over to the window.

"God is crying," I said softly to myself, hoping no one heard, as I watched the drops hit the glass. "I feel he's giving me a signal—that he knows my situation and is here with me."

44

These personal conversations gave me comfort. Rain is a cleanser, and my body certainly needed that.

- *Cancer patients often feel a closer link with a higher power or spiritual being. It's reassuring to have that special relationship with someone or something greater than yourself, whom you can talk to and confide in. Try it and see if it works in your own way and your own time.*

I went back to my seat and waited for my flight to be called. Suddenly, a Continental ticket agent appeared out of nowhere.

"Excuse me Mrs. Parker, we're moving you to a different seat on the plane," he said gently.

"That's fine with me as long as it's not too far back," I replied, looking rather morose with eyes red from tearing.

Like many people newly diagnosed with a serious illness, I had spent some alone time crying.

Several months later, I found out that Continental Airlines upgrades M.D. Anderson cancer patients, if there's room on the flight. I was one of the lucky ones. I looked at my seat number as I neared the gate for boarding. 14A had been changed to 4B. I burst into tears of joy. My emotions were running high.

"I don't know how to thank you," I said wiping the tears away.

"You don't have to thank me," the man replied. "Just get well. I'm a cancer survivor myself." I stood right up and gave this perfect stranger a big hug. He had changed a negative into a positive just by moving my seat.

- *You can change the outlook of a cancer patient by doing something special. Cancer patients need to feel that they are still deserving of surprises that bring them joy and hope.*

Was this an omen? Were good things about to happen for me too? Would I be offered a second chance at life? I wasn't sure, but I knew that I'd never forget that gate attendant's gesture as I boarded the early morning plane to Houston.

All the way to Texas, I thought about my decision to head west. After all, it was my life. Even though George, John, and Amy thought it was the best place for me, the cancer patient has to agree. Rationalizing how much I'd already learned from the esteemed doctors at NYU Medical Center and Memorial Sloan- Kettering, who would have willingly treated me, I knew that without having family or a home near the hospital, it just didn't seem feasible.

Knowing that we would have a hard time finding a place to rent in pricy New York City, especially with two English setters in tow, the best decision was to head to Houston and meet a Dr. André Goy.

- *When a cancer patient has made the decision where to go for the best treatment, the stress starts to diminish and the fighting spirit moves in.*

As I crossed the country, I had plenty of time for reflection. My mind darted back to when I married George, in 1963. It brought a smile to my face. How innocent I was back then! The culinary creations I prepared as a nineteen-year-old bride included scrambled eggs, grilled-cheese and tomato sandwiches, and hot chocolate. Everything else was prepared on our new Rotobroil 400, a shower gift from George's mom. In his view, my best culinary talent was one dessert that he adored—a chocolate devil's food cake with a white maple syrup icing.

My mom taught me the family recipe in our Vermont kitchen when I was a little girl. You had to use just the right formula. I could almost smell the maple syrup frosting when it came to me. Coming to M.D. Anderson would be like baking a perfect cake. One would choose the ingredients, mix them precisely, place them very carefully in a well-greased pan, and voilà—forty-five minutes later, a luscious devil's food cake would materialize, waiting to be frosted!

The smile turned into a grin as I wondered whether Dr. André Goy might be the "French pastry chef" who would know when, where, and how to turn my body back into that perfectly baked confection. All my hopes and dreams would be with this doctor, whom I'd never met. Fantasy and hope were two intangibles that I relied on heavily to help me as I crossed into the Lone Star State.

When I landed in Texas, I was feeling a little drained after the long trip from New York. John was waiting at the airport and whisked me off with my single piece of carry-on luggage.

He and his wife owned a wonderful new home in a northwest suburb of Houston. The neighborhood was young, vibrant, and alive, with children and dogs playing outside on manicured lawns. I was soon ensconced in their guest room on the second floor. It was all white wicker and had its own bathroom.

• *When a cancer patient decides to go away from home for treatment, a close relative is often the best choice because it is the most like home.*

I even tried to forget the real reason I was there and put on my lipstick and blush as if I were going shopping. John would soon teach me the route to M.D. Anderson, some thirty miles south through heavy city traffic.

John had warned me that Houston was huge, just like Texas. I had no idea what he meant, but I soon found out. There were multitudes of highways to get on and off, and there were real "cowboys" on the road.

At this point, the adventuresome spirit in me seemed to have waned. Although usually fearless when it came to driving, I was feeling a bit apprehensive. "It's easy Mom," he said optimistically, "You'll get used to this in no time." Was he kidding?

Forty-five minutes later, we were in south central Houston. John had reserved a room for one night at the Rotary House Marriott, so that I'd be right across the street from the cancer center for my first appointment at 7 A.M. the following morning. There was a glass-enclosed bridge connecting the hotel and the hospital and a riot of flowers. I began to sing "There's a Yellow Rose in Texas."

• *Singing was my antidote for being afraid. Concentrating on the words and music took away the fear. Immersing yourself in music may help you too.*

"I think I'm going to like it here," I said, hoping to dispel any apprehension I was feeling and not wanting to be a burden. No cancer patient ever does. We checked in and John walked me to my room. George had returned to South Carolina and was driving our car and the dogs eleven hundred miles to the west. I hugged John, and the more I thanked him the more he told me, "It was nothing!"

Rush hour was beginning and I assured him that I could handle my first encounter with M.D. Anderson alone. He wasn't so sure. Finally convinced, he disappeared into Houston traffic.

Thinking about the kind of person he had grown into, I took a moment to be a proud mom. My eyes were blinded with tears from nowhere as I watched him fade in the distance, hoping we'd have good news and I'd be his mom for a long time to come.

Starting this new adventure in life, I walked back into the hotel, heading to an area called "Patient Relations," in the back of the lobby. "How nice of them to realize that guests might need some orientation in such a big complex," I thought to myself. Sitting alone, I watched a ten-minute video about cancer. But instead of feeling reassured, I became frightened because there were so many cancers, so much to learn. This was a topic I still didn't want to know anything about.

- *Cancer patients are often in denial. It is common and you will come to the realization, as I did, that although it's not the best thing to have, we can conquer our fears and fight the enemy head on.*

Wiping away some new tears, I proceeded into the "Resource Center" and picked up a booklet on lymphoma and Hodgkin's disease. After perusing it, I began to cry. I wasn't ready to read it; all I wanted was to go home. The booklets were published by the American Cancer Society to help educate patients and their families. Topics discussed included the possibility of surviving the original cancer but later developing a secondary one as a result of the radiation or chemotherapy treatments. I wasn't ready to hear that. I just wanted my life back the way it used to be.

I called George on the cell phone.

"Come and get me," I sobbed. "This is more than I ever bargained for. The pamphlets here talk about the possibilities of more cancer in a few years."

George was calming as always. "Give this a chance. You haven't even been to the cancer center yet. It's going to be fine, Sharon, and I'm on my way."

- *Being alone at this time may not have been the best decision. But cancer patients need to feel that they can survive while still handling whatever is thrown their way. Self-confidence builds on each little success and makes reaching the goal of becoming cancer-free that much easier to achieve.*

- *Positive reinforcement is important for every patient. Make sure you get it from someone who'll be there for you no matter what.*

One of the rare qualities I consistently saw in George, giving me renewed hope, was that he always saw the good in everything.

"It all happens for a purpose," he had said repeatedly. "Even your sister-in-law Sandy says, 'Whenever you get lemons, you make lemonade'." Now I smile just thinking about it. It's a phrase worth remembering.

"OK," I said, "I won't sit up in the lobby worrying all night." Attempting to make me feel better, he used positive reinforcement as a tool, and it worked.

"Have a safe trip, but please hurry."

I started to think and plan as I walked back to my room. Was it too late? Did we catch this in time? "God, please help me," I whispered. "I need you now."

7

M.D. Anderson's Dr. Goy

I believe, for every drop of rain that falls,
A flower grows...
I believe that somewhere in the darkest night,
A candle glows...
I believe for everyone who goes astray,
Someone will come, to show the way...

from "I Believe"

The friendly "good morning" hotel operator rang and woke me from a deep sleep. Dressing quickly, I drank some cranberry juice and headed over to the lymphoma clinic across the enclosed glass bridge that led from the hotel to Dr. Goy's office on the eighth floor of the outpatient building.

I couldn't believe how tremendous the M.D. Anderson Cancer Center was. Doctors and nurses were coming and going throughout the hallways and offices. So many foreign languages were heard, and the information signs were easily seen. Patients were here from near and far and like me, each one of them was hoping to be cured.

The elevator stopped on every floor, and it was hard not to notice the signs for different parts of the body: Breast, Colon, Brain and Spine, Head and Neck, Bone, Blood, Gastrointestinal. Everything was so specialized. Finally, I reached the eighth floor: Myeloma, non-Hodgkin's lymphoma, and Hodgkin's lymphoma to the left; Leukemia to the right.

Lymphoma. Just seeing the word sent a chill through my body. My heart was pounding as I took a deep breath.

"Don't be so nervous," I heard myself saying, *"You have nothing to fear but fear itself."* Thank you, President Roosevelt, for those words of wisdom. "Onward, Forward, Positive," I said quietly to myself as I walked briskly toward my destination.

That particular walk seemed to go on forever, as I passed waiting rooms for other types of cancer. It was suddenly obvious to me who the patients were; once again, they were the ones, with few exceptions, who weren't smiling while waiting for their appointments. The friends and relatives I saw were chatting and asking questions, but many patients seemed somber. Perhaps, it was because cancer can be overwhelming. Many had lost their hair due to chemotherapy, while others had obvious scars or bandages somewhere on their bodies.

"Smile," I heard myself say. "You have Hodgkin's and you are going to deal with it in the most positive way possible." A broad smile emerged as I sat down to wait my turn.

- *I wondered how many other people talked to themselves; I do, and especially when there's no one around, it's helpful. Sometimes I can be two people, the one who asks the questions and the one who gives me the answers. Whatever works for you is what you should do.*

There was a large waiting room with lots of upholstered chairs. A television was already turned on, and tropical fish were swimming in their tanks. Two receptionists were busy with patients waiting to see a number of different doctors. In this area, all of the doctors were lymphoma specialists. I saw my doctor's name listed and prayed silently that he could help me. It was my first appointment with Dr. Goy, and to be honest, I was as nervous as a long-tailed cat in a room full of rocking chairs.

This man held my future in the palm of his hand, and I was thankful that he came so highly recommended by an outstanding doctor in New York. Dr. Zelenetz had picked Dr. Goy without hesitation.

- *You need to go to the most qualified oncologist you can find through the Internet, recommendation, or your own experience.*

While I was filling out yet another long questionnaire and waiting patiently in my chair, a young volunteer in a pink coat came over and offered everyone coffee or tea. It was a nice gesture, but I declined. I was happy to be there but very unhappy with my cancer diagnosis.

A cheerful nurse called out my name. She led me to a chair and took my blood pressure, pulse, weight, and temperature. I took off my shoes. I didn't want to weigh one ounce more than I had to. Temperature 97.6, blood pressure 110/70, weight 127 pounds. She asked many questions as I sat in the examining room. I had plenty to tell and didn't stop until the door opened and a man in a long white coat walked in.

From the moment Dr. Goy entered the room, I felt his strong presence and warm personality. After the initial examination, he informed me about all of my test results. He confirmed the initial diagnosis and gently indicated the presence of an additional, totally unrelated cancer, called metastatic papillary follicular thyroid carcinoma. This seemed impossible. My hand went immediately to my neck. I felt no lumps and my pulse quickened. Was I doomed?

"Why didn't they see this in New York, Dr. Goy?"

"The reason is simple," he replied. "When a biopsy is performed, it's broken into three sections, A, B, and C. Only the first two sections were made into slides, stained, and analyzed. No thyroid cancer was evident. Our pathologist asked that the C block be sent to us unstained. NYU Medical Center obliged, and our doctors found a tiny focus in the new specimen. However, I don't want you to worry about it now, Mrs. Parker. We'll treat the Hodgkin's first and address the thyroid cancer later."

After listening to him for a few minutes, my fear and trepidation gave way to a calm reality. I was in deep trouble, but I regained my composure and felt that if anyone could come up with the right answers, it was he. I had absolutely no symptoms of thyroid cancer. But no matter how much I disagreed, it didn't seem to matter.

It was a lot to digest in one meeting, but Dr. Goy's positive approach was reassuring. Curing two cancers in one body would not be easy. However, he seemed extremely confident that they could make me well again, and that confidence is contagious.

- *Confidence is one ingredient you need to beat cancer. Finding the doctor who can instill it is the key.*

Now I'd listen to everything he would tell me to do in order to rid my body of the cancers. He would send me downstairs to a thyroid specialist, Dr. Steven Sherman, and together they would map out my treatment plan.

Perhaps I was born under a lucky star, because Dr. Goy turned out to be much more than just an oncologist. He was brilliant, positive, caring, and extremely well educated. My instinct was at work once again, assuring me that I had been put in the hands of a unique physician: I knew I couldn't have asked for more.

At the time, I never considered how others diagnosed with cancer felt about their doctors. What I did know was that Dr. Goy made me believe that, together, we would fight the cancers that were making a home in my body. The intensity in his eyes and his warm smile coupled with his positive approach didn't hurt one bit either!

Perhaps the most reassuring aspect for me was Dr. Goy's passion for the most updated treatments. Research was an essential part of his everyday life. He was a leader in clinical trials and in the development of new techniques. I'*d*

*soon learn that he was a great believer in consulting with
other experts worldwide. He shared his ideas and listened to
the views of others before making final decisions.*

We said our good-byes, and although I was unable to
remember the long name of the second cancer, I was calmer
knowing that Dr. Goy would be there for me a hundred percent. His unique combination of skills gave me the courage
and strength I needed to forge ahead. I thought about the
other cancer patients I saw in the waiting rooms and hoped
they would come away feeling as I did. It would make all
the difference in the world for me. From that day on, I'd
learn to appreciate every moment of life on this earth.

* *Cancer is a rude awakening for all of us, so don't let the little troubles that plague each of us grow into big problems.
We learn, sometimes the hard way, that every day we are
on this earth is a great gift. We can't waste our time concentrating on the negatives. Instead, we need to get a grip
and follow the best plan for optimal results. Some of us
may be cured, others may be in remission, but new therapies developed by cancer experts are being tried every
day.*

I have no doubt that because of the Dr. Goys of the
world, we will be cured and be here to help others survive.

8

The Lady from Johannesburg

Grab your coat and get your hat
Leave your worries on the doorstep
Life can be so sweet
On the sunny side of the street
from "Sunny Side of the Street"

May 15, 2002

The Houston traffic and I were beginning to understand each other. Whenever you move to a new place, it takes time to adjust and learn the ropes. In the beginning, days before treatment began, I was doing just that.

John and Chrissy had welcomed me into their new home. Though married just five years, they invited me to stay with them for the six-month treatment period. It was wonderful to feel loved, but their beautiful house was in the very northwest tip of Houston; the hospital was right in the middle of the south central section of town. In some cities that might not matter. But who knew Houston was so huge? It went on for miles and miles. Incredible! Regardless, I was glad to be with my family, and John reminded me to leave plenty of extra time for the drive.

George was flying back and forth from Charleston and would soon be able to stay in Texas for longer periods. He was hoping to work out of the Lone Star state, on a more permanent basis if his company would allow, and they did.

"This house is too far from the hospital," I remember him saying, after the first few days of commuting during morning rush-hour congestion, as we crawled to M.D. Anderson for more tests. "You need to be closer to the hospital in case of an emergency."

I agreed. I just didn't know where to start, or even if I could summon the energy, to look for a place to live.

Later that same day, George drove around a residential area near the hospital. The last thing I felt like doing was house hunting. But perhaps he was right.

"You need to be close to the hospital in case of an emergency, that's what Andy Zelnetz said in New York," he reminded me.

I thought about the money it would cost to rent. It was already overwhelming to think about the astronomical medical bills, which soon would be mounting.

"Thank God for insurance," I said aloud, not having any idea how long it would take for the payments to begin.

We drove onto a very nice residential street, quite by accident. George made a left and then a right, having no real idea where we were going. Suddenly, there appeared a "for sale" sign in front of a gray rambling house with navy shutters on a large corner lot. Outside, by the curb, was a little stand holding the sales information.

"Shall we stop to get an idea of how much homes cost around here?" I queried.

"Good idea," he replied gently, "but I don't think we want to buy anything."

As I slowly got out of the car, at 6 P.M., it was still light in Houston. Suddenly, as if it were planned, a blonde-haired lady appeared at the front door.

"Would you like to see my house?" she asked invitingly, with an accent that I assumed to be British.

"She must be from England," I whispered. "Shall we go have a look?"

"Absolutely," George responded. "How unusual: she doesn't even know us and yet she asked us in!"

"Houston must be the friendliest place in the world," I replied, not having any idea whom we had accidentally encountered.

"How do you do?" my husband said with an outstretched hand. "I'm George Parker, and this is my wife Sharon. We're here from South Carolina, seeing what's available."

"I'm an M.D. Anderson cancer patient," just tumbled out of my mouth. It took us both by surprise.

"I'm Dr. Ruth Katz, a professor of pathology at M.D. Anderson," she casually replied with an ingratiating smile that put us both at ease.

There was a sudden gasp of amazement from the two of us which couldn't be muffled.

There were five million people in Houston. And there we were standing in front of a house owned by a doctor from the same cancer center that held my future in its grasp. "Where are you from?" I asked, quickly regaining my composure.

"I'm originally from Johannesburg, South Africa," she replied.

She certainly has charisma, I thought to myself.

"Do you know my doctor, André Goy?" I inquired.

"Oh, yes; I know him very well. We're involved in research projects together."

"Outstanding," I replied, encouraged by the coincidence.

"Sit down," she offered graciously. "I'll get you some tea and we can talk."

George looked so relieved. I could see the tension leave his drawn face. Here we were in a new city, in a stranger's house, but somehow it was as if we were meant to be all together.

"I'm very impressed with Dr. Goy," I remarked, hoping to elicit a response.

"He's one of the best in the world at what he does; and he is a man with heart," she replied candidly.

• *Every cancer patient wants to feel reassured that the right decision has been made as far as choosing the most qualified oncologist.*

"I feel that already," I answered. "He has a positive spirit and so much knowledge, it put me at ease right away."

"Don't you worry; you've got the right man."

"I can't believe I have two cancers," I continued.

"Hodgkin's is the best kind to have," she said without hesitating.

"I also have papillary thyroid cancer," I said unabashedly, forgetting the rest of the name and a meningioma sitting on my occipital lobe.

"There's a lot we can do, and I'll be seeing your slides," she offered reassuringly.

"WOW!" I thought, "God must be watching over me right now." We took a tour of her house and found out the price.

"We're really not sure what to do," George continued. "We have a home in Boca Raton, Florida, and I work in South Carolina. Right now, we're staying with our son John in Northwest Houston."

"Oh, that's too far away for Sharon, with all the traffic," the concerned doctor replied.

"That's what I thought," George quickly agreed, not knowing where this would lead.

"I have an idea. I've built a townhouse just five minutes from here. I plan to move into it myself. But you go look at it: if you like it, you can live there. It's brand new."

I couldn't believe my ears. After all the cancer news we had, could something this good be happening to us? "Let's go have a look," George urged, as Dr. Katz handed us the keys.

The townhouse was beautiful. There it sat, three stories high, five minutes from M.D. Anderson; sparkling clean, with a granite kitchen, moldings, wood floors, and a little terrace. "Oh, it's perfect," we said in unison.

There was a bedroom on the ground floor and another on the third. I'd have a choice, I thought, depending on whether I had the strength to climb the stairs after chemotherapy. The townhouse was almost ready to move into, missing only a washer, dryer, and refrigerator. "We'll, take it," I heard George say gleefully.

"Even if we can't afford it," I piped in.

- *Paying rent for a place for a cancer patient to live might sound extravagant. But when a life is on the line, the physical and emotional well-being of the patient needs to be factored in and can make the difference in a positive outcome.*

We signed a rental agreement that evening.

"We have two seven-year-old English setters," I added, hoping against hope that she was a dog lover as well.

"You can bring them to the townhouse; they'll help you get well again," she answered with a grin.

A smile as big as the state of Texas spread across my face, as tears of joy fell from my eyes. We would be near the hospital and the doctors, who would do their very best to eliminate all cancer from my body. Everything was fitting into place, and coming to Texas was surely the right decision.

- *Cancer patients need to know that there are giving people out there who will help if they just know the circumstances. Don't ever be afraid to ask.*

The next morning we bought a bed, refrigerator, and a washer-dryer. Hearing that I had cancer, Conn's appliance store in Northwest Houston went out of their way to deliver everything as soon as possible. Again I thought: "Houston, what a city! The people are unbelievably caring." I witnessed it first hand over and over again: Perfect strangers outstretching their hands to help their fellow man. It's a lesson we can all remember. This act of generosity and kindness by a woman we had never met before was a tremendous boost to our morale. We were almost like newlyweds again, and even if we maxed out the credit cards, we would find a way.

9

What to Do, When You're Told You've Got Two!

Que sera, sera,
Whatever will be, will be;
The future's not ours to see.
Que sera, sera...

from "Que Sera, Sera"

Things that come in twos are usually reason to celebrate. However, hearing that you have two unrelated cancers is not something most people are prepared to handle.

Any person struck with one cancer has a full plate. It takes great skill and courage to tell another human being that they have more; especially when no one initially thought there was anything seriously wrong in the first place. Remembering how Dr. Goy was able to break the news in the most positive way possible must have given me that much needed determination to go on.

Perhaps it was the direction and professionalism of Dr. Goy and Dr. Sherman, the endocrinologist who became the other part of the healing team, that put me at ease and gave me the ability to focus on the cure.

Dr. Steven Sherman, a senior endocrinologist at M.D. Anderson, was the man with the plan for the thyroid gland. When he saw me after having a consult with Dr. Goy, it was agreed that the lymphoma needed to be eliminated first because it was more acute and the most serious and significant cancer in my body.

62

Dr. Sherman put me on a drug to stop the pituitary gland from producing any more thyroid-stimulating hormone (TSH); this would stop the thyroid from sending new malignant cells out to multiply in my system. Every day on waking, I'd take a pill of synthetic thyroid hormone (Synthroid) designed to do this job.

I'd agreed to all the tests and sonograms Dr. Sherman requested; everything was working according to plan.

* *Being an active participant in the treatment of two cancers requires a positive focus and provides plenty of new information to absorb.*

Like most cancer patients, I've learned more than I ever thought I wanted to know, but I find it interesting and hope that a cure will be found for everyone. Even remembering the name "metastatic papillary follicular variant thyroid carcinoma" deserves an award, and I'm grateful that I don't have a more aggressive form.

If surgery is ever indicated, a surgeon will remove the thyroid gland. Several weeks later, a dose of radiation therapy (with radioactive isotope I-131) would be necessary and administered orally so as to kill any thyroid cells that might still be hiding in my body.

Only Dr. Sherman and the radiologists will be able to decide whether this cancer has gone to sleep for good. I look forward to having it checked every six months and watching out for any symptoms. Hoarseness, coughing, or swollen lymph nodes in my neck would mandate an immediate call to them. Meanwhile, I concentrate on getting stronger every day, feeling that God is watching over me.

10

Lessons in Life

Oh! It's a good day, for singin' a song,
An' it's a good day for movin' along,
Yes, it's a good day, how could anything go wrong?
A good day from mornin' 'till night!
from "It's A Good Day"

May 18, 2002 A.M.

We were just getting used to the new townhouse and finding our way around the city when the day arrived for Chemo 101. Thinking academically, I decided to pretend that I was going to a college chemistry seminar and every two weeks would change the number of the class until the required twelve were reached.

A strange combination of excitement and fright filled my mind as we drove to the cancer center at 6:45 A.M. It was quiet, with only a few people milling about the huge complex at such an early hour. My schedule didn't begin until 8 A.M., but like a good student, I wanted to be sure I had arrived on time and gotten my bearings.

George and I were alone in the elevator, as we headed to the third floor for blood and urine tests. Suddenly, he grabbed my hand.

"You're going to be fine," he said tenderly.

- *A caregiver carries his own tremendous burden, keeping up not only his own spirits but those of the patient as well.*

My eyes filled with tears as I kissed his hand.

"I do hope you're right," I replied softly.

The waiting room was all but empty, with only fifty chairs waiting for patients and a young receptionist seated behind a large desk.

"Good morning," I said politely, "I'm Sharon Lee Parker, patient number 379421."

"I'm sorry Mrs. Parker, but there's a block on your account and no blood can be drawn until it's removed," she said contritely.

I looked up at George incredulously. "What does this mean?"

"Perhaps they want some money," he replied in a subdued manner.

• *Cancer care is becoming more expensive and, for most of us, this is an important issue. Cancer patients must be prepared and aware that the costs can be overwhelming and that they may need help from an outside source if they are not adequately insured.*

We were directed to the eighth floor to see a financial counselor, but no one was there; it was too early. At precisely 8 A.M., the clinic began to buzz with activity as the staff arrived, and George was ushered into a private office. I elected to stay out in the waiting room, concentrating instead on the tropical fish and listening to the music of the rain pelting the windows.

"Think happy thoughts," I said to myself. "Everything will work out."

George soon reappeared and asked for my checkbook. Thank heavens I had remembered to put one in my bag.

"They want the medical insurance deductible and co-pay."

"How much?" I asked, having no idea what was coming next.

"$6,500," he said flatly.

All I could say was, "WOW!" I wasn't sure if I had that much in the account but George had wisely secured the funds that would enable me to proceed.

A few minutes later, we were back on track, heading to have my blood and urine checked. I was amazed at how crowded the waiting room had become. So many people had cancer! I had a funny feeling that my veins were not about to cooperate with anyone, given the way the day had started.

Sure enough, the skilled phlebotomist had a difficult time getting my blood to flow. The first vein was stubborn and flatly refused to cooperate. She wasn't about to give up, however, and finally found one that was willing to oblige. After a quick trip to the bathroom, I realized that on that day, leaving a urine sample was a lot easier than a blood sample.

- *A gentle reminder to drink lots of water before blood tests was great advice. It pumps up the veins and makes drawing blood a cinch, with just a little pinch.*

We hurried back to see Dr. Goy. Before any chemotherapy could begin, he would make certain I was healthy enough for the treatment. My blood counts had to be checked each time to make sure that they were at acceptable levels. When I finally received the go-ahead for Chemo 101, Dr. Goy asked, "Would you care to participate in a study?"

"What kind of study?" I queried.

"We're trying to obtain some cells from the lymph nodes of lymphoma patients for lab studies on a current project."

"I'll help," was my immediate response, as I looked to George for approval.

We headed down to the Fine Needle Aspiration Clinic at the far end of the cancer center.

"Will this hurt?" I asked the researcher waiting to begin.

"No, it shouldn't. It's just a fine needle aspiration."

Once again, my body wouldn't cooperate. The lymph node in my neck couldn't easily be found and, after four attempts and a dose of tranquillizer, she gave up. Was it my rather loud wail or the fact that the tiny node may have been hiding behind a muscle in my neck? As a large ice pack was gently placed at the point of needle insertion, all I knew was that I didn't help the study.

As we walked slowly back toward the lymphoma clinic, I felt sedated and my ego was deflated. I put my pocket book down on a hallway chair while George helped me on with a jacket to cover my chilled body. We then continued walking from the green zone through the blue zone, and to the rose zone without saying much. All of a sudden, it hit me...my purse was still sitting on that chair, a quarter mile away.

"My bag," I cried as George turned and raced back, but it was nowhere to be seen. Who would believe that this was happening on my first chemo day? Later it was found by a security guard with everything intact except for the money George had given me that morning.

- *That day taught me many valuable lessons. Always remember to check with the financial office the day before to make sure the account is up to date. Drinking lots of water will help your blood flow for all of the day's blood tests. If you experience any pain, the doctors and nurses will want to know. There is often a medication to solve the problem. Finally, never bring more that $25 in cash to the hospital. It's easy to lose track of things, and the last thing you need is more stress. Perhaps the most valuable lesson of the day was to remember to keep it all in perspective.*

What really mattered was whether the chemotherapy would start to kill off the terrorists that had taken my body hostage. That question would be answered one way or the other through the long treatment process, which was to begin in just a few hours.

- *One final note: Ask for a copy of every result for the tests you take. Keep your own notebook for future reference. You have a right to the results, but they are not always offered. Speak up and don't be shy. One day you'll be very glad you did.*

ABVD Day
Grey skies are gonna clear up
Put on a happy face;
Brush all the clouds and cheer up
Put on a happy face...
from "Put On A Happy Face"

May 18, 2002 P.M.

My chemo nurse, Christine, was young, beautiful, and from the Philippines. She was soon to be married and was having her reception at a Marriott. I told her about my son John, who managed a Houston Marriott. She said she'd call him if she had any questions. We were like a mother and daughter having a lovely chat as she skillfully inserted the needle into my arm. Four chemo drugs—doxorubicin (Adriamycin), bleomycin, dacarbazine, and vinblastine—were soon delivered into my body via that vein.

"Two of these are very powerful," she said. "They're called vesicants and they can be irritating to your veins. Please let me know if it hurts too much." How kind of her, I thought to myself. I had never heard of these drugs before and was surprised I could even pronounce them. It was simpler just to call them ABVD.

I was curious about the saline solution she used after each drug was fully administered.

"Think of it as a bath for your veins," she said brightly.

Whatever she did, I knew I felt better. Her kind, gentle, and learned ways fostered my confidence in the prescribed treatment plan. I left Chemo 101 behind with a smile and was able to drive home with George as the passenger.

When I saw him a few days later, Dr. Goy was thrilled with the outcome of my first treatment. It was obvious by the smile on his face.

"You'll be fine," he insisted, as he listened to my chest and checked me over carefully.

I was a new woman.

"I stayed up all night in the bathroom and let all the poison out of me. I must have drunk at least ten half-liter bottles of water."

"Good," he said, "The more water, the better, and ride your stationary bike to help keep your strength up."

"Oh I will," I said enthusiastically. "I even took the antinausea medication, but I wasn't sure if, at $39 a pill, I really needed it."

"You'll see in time," he said. "Just keep them handy."

"One little pill, called Zofran (ondansetron), which you put on your tongue, dissolves in a few seconds—it's unbelievable, it costs so much," I continued.

"There's no generic equivalent," he added, "and until there is, this can be a lifesaver. Did you notice your urine turned pink?"

"That was a big surprise, but the nurse told me to expect it, so I wasn't worried."

"Good," he said, "You'll be fine. See you in two weeks."

I wanted to give him a hug. I liked him so much already. His eyes lit up, his smile was genuine. I was one lucky lady to have a doctor who really cared and showed it.

When I left M.D. Anderson that day, I went shopping. I stopped off at the Whole Foods Market where I bought lanolin for my lips, a natural shampoo for my now precious hair, which was still clinging to my scalp, and fresh flowers for my kitchen table, along with organically grown fruits and vegetables. Next, I was off to the neighboring linen mart for a "bed in a bag" quilt and sheet set for my newly acquired mattress. What more could a girl want?

All of a sudden my nose felt stuffy. Was my white blood cell count dropping already due to the chemotherapy?

- *Cancer patients need to remember that their white count can drop to immune-compromised low levels and that serious sources of infection should be avoided. I found it comforting to steer clear of large crowds and people coughing for the duration of chemotherapy. I didn't want to take a chance of getting sick and having to stop my treatments. Ask your doctors what they recommend. Perhaps at some point the drugs filgrastim (Neupogen) and epoetin alfa (Procrit) may be prescribed in order to keep your blood count in the normal range and your body ready for the fight of its life.*

Eventually George would bring me a Boehm porcelain flower from our home. I had been collecting them for years. They are still handmade and look better than real ones because they never wilt.

Part II

11

Living Life to the Fullest

Would you like to ride in my beautiful balloon?
Would you like to glide in my beautiful balloon?
We could fly among the stars together, you and I.
For we can fly!
from "Up Up and Away"

Thinking philosophically, how can we be expected to "enjoy life," when the thoughts of having cancer and all of its consequences are subtle reminders that our days of carefree living are a thing of the past? For example, it becomes a daunting task to remain in the mainstream of life while trying to avoid everyone with a bad cough or cold. Perhaps I was being overly cautious, but I wanted to do everything possible to remain healthy. It reminds me of the tightrope walker in the circus. Life becomes a balancing act. How do you participate and still protect yourself while going through the months of chemotherapy?

- *One solution is to surround yourself with those people who understand the situation and who build your spirit by not making a big deal out of any changes you feel are necessary. Protecting your health and well-being is the first priority now.*

Dr. Goy often said to live my life as normally as possible but to use common sense, especially during those days when my white count was dropping. Not wanting to become reclusive but still concerned about being cured without unnecessary complications, what could I do?

- *Look for creative ways to make each day as complete and fulfilling as possible.*

- *The television, the Internet, and the radio are instant company and can fill anyone's living space with another voice.*

Reading, walking, singing, listening to music, and playing the piano fill my alone time and reward me with a sense of accomplishment. But what can people do when they can't think of a hobby or are more pessimistic about their outcome?

The answer is complex, because each of us comes to cancer with a different set of feelings and emotions. Most of us want to be part of the mainstream even if we're dealing with chemotherapy, surgery, or radiation. We take a "time out" and then bounce back, grateful for the life we have. For others it's not so easy, because the emotional toll is greater. Some of my cancer pals talked to therapists. Others needed medication to help them over the hurdles. For me the best treatment was conscientiously focusing on the idea that I'd be fine and do everything that Dr. Goy suggested in order to get well.

- *It's optimism versus pessimism. Surrounding yourself with positive people—whether on the phone, the Internet, or in person—is a reassuring tonic every day.*

Some well-meaning people may startle you with, "Oh, I don't know how you're coping," or "I'd kill myself if I had what you have."

- *Destructive conversations, no matter how well-meaning, can change your attitude and your outcome, so let them go.*

I find that when I'm strong, I can handle almost anything that comes my way; but when you're fighting cancer, what another person says or does takes on new meanings.

- *Positive people, positive thoughts, and good old-fashioned common sense will help us heal and look to the future. Surround yourself with love and caring and keep that "emotional raincoat" handy. When you're hit with negative comments, put it on to keep those contrary statements at bay.*

Since there were two weeks between chemo treatments, I decided to try to do something interesting every day. My recovery was helped by concentrating on enjoying the great pleasures that life offers, including the sun, moon, birds, squirrels, chipmunks, flowers, stars, and majestic trees.

As part of my cure, I'd often sit on my tiny terrace, in the back of the townhouse, drinking fresh bottled water or sipping green tea, taking in all that God had created. Dr. Goy repeatedly reminded me of the importance of exercise. Riding a stationary bicycle each day was mandatory. It gave me more energy and a feeling of well-being. Remembering to avoid exposure to direct sunlight while undergoing chemotherapy, due to increased photosensitivity, was another new rule

Sometimes doing something out of the ordinary adds a little spice to your life. One cloudy day I walked to a Thrifty Car Rental agency, just a few blocks away. Spotting a shiny new red Chrysler Sebring convertible, I decided it was just waiting for me. After telling my daughter-in-law Chrissy that red was a policeman's favorite target, I rented it for the week. Now, I'd have my own sporty car, and it did the trick. I felt like a new woman.

Parking at a nearby Talbot's store, I bought a Bristol blue wide-brimmed straw hat to protect my face from the hazy Houston sun. I took a spin around town and felt more like the old happy me every minute. I remember that Dr. Goy had said "There will be good days and some not-so-good days, but you will be fine."

Well, that day I was fine, and I was going to enjoy every minute of it!

When my sister Ellen called from Florida that night, it was nearing 10 P.M. and I was simply too tired to talk. She was on a different schedule and showed concern, but I needed to sleep, and going to bed early was part of my healing routine. Learning to think of *me* first was a new experience. Ellen left a message that she wanted to visit soon, but I wasn't ready. I needed time to adjust to new schedules and to learn to cope with everything that had become vital in my fight for survival. The visits would come later.

* *Washing your hands often during the day and keeping your fingers away from your mouth to keep germs at bay are important considerations I found well worth remembering. Pesticides, insecticides, and other people's serious infections, such as chickenpox, can be a real concern. Stay away from them and use common sense when you feel at risk. When flying on a commercial airline, ask your doctor if a mask is advisable; it may feel like Halloween but you'll get used to it. When your neutrophil count is less than 0.5, your oncologist may tell you that you are at a higher risk of infection and give you specific instructions.*

Every day I took a multivitamin, as well as other prescribed medications, to make sure my body rebuilt a strong immune system. Even my diet needed to be modified. According to doctors' orders, my new meal plan included some fat and lots of protein. The nutritionist at M.D. Anderson spoke about the many ways of maintaining my weight.

• *During chemotherapy, appetites can disappear with the onset of mouth sores, caused by reactions to specific drugs.*

Weight loss may interfere with recovery, so anything that tasted good and soothing was added to my menu options.

• *It is a good idea to make an appointment with a cancer center dietitian for some ideas on exactly what to eat.*

How I remember George going off to Randall's Supermarket and purchasing three pints of Ben and Jerry's ice cream, in a variety of flavors. I dug right into delicious Vanilla Swirl, thrilled to finally be able to indulge myself without feeling guilty. There were positives going through chemotherapy, after all. However, *moderation is a key to everything in life,* including Vanilla Swirl.

• *Becoming acclimated and accepting the hand you've been dealt are other positive steps all cancer patients can take.*

• *Letting your spirit soar whenever something good happens makes both the cancer patient and the caregiver feel that progress is being made. Hope, an intangible that is contagious, can help lead to the results you're looking for.*

I needed to smile. Admittedly sometimes it was forced, but I did it anyway until it became second nature. *Laughter became as important as exercise.* Watching comedies or reading something funny can change brain chemistry. It works for both the cancer patient and the caregiver.

- *Even if you think you have nothing to laugh about, do it anyway. It costs nothing and the outcome can bring big rewards.*

- *Embracing life with all of its pluses and opening the window to "let the sunshine in" is the perfect antidote for negative emotions.*

Getting well and back into the main stream of life is the wish of every cancer patient. Some days may be rough, but we have to be tough and become a part of the healing team that will lead us to recovery.

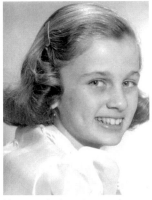

I began singing at an early age. At age 10, I won a radio talent contest, which led to my first recording contract.

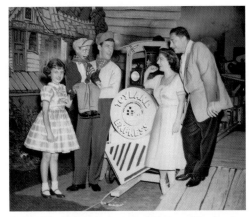

As I child, I appeared on the TV show, "Toyland Express." To my right is Paul Winchell, my agent Sally Pearl, and the orchestra leader, Mel Gold.

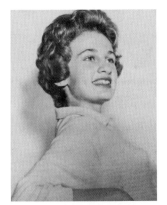

I am pictured here as "Suzy Star." I signed my next recording contract with ABC Paramount Records, at age 17.

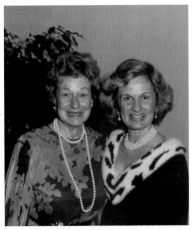

My mother Cecilia was my best friend and my mentor. She died suddenly while I was undergoing treatment.

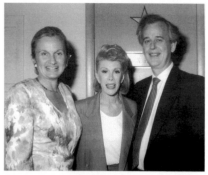

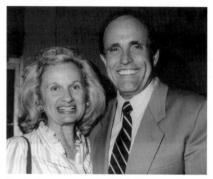

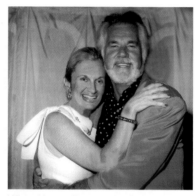

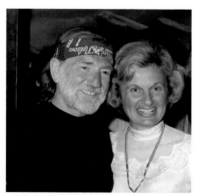

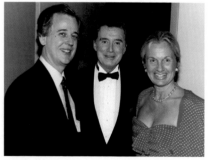

Comedienne Joan Rivers, here with me and George, made us laugh many times when she played at the Concord Hotel. She is a real success story.

When Kenny Rogers played at the Concord, he sang my favorite, "You Decorated My Life."

Rudy Guiliani attended a Sons of Italy Convention at the hotel. He is one of the brightest politicians I've ever met.

Singer Willie Nelson arrived in his famous bus. Meeting him was a real joy.

Regis Philbin, here with me and George, was always an audience favorite when he came to shows at the Concord.

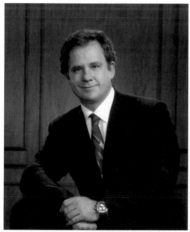

Dr. Andre Goy was the lymphoma specialist whom I credit with saving my life.

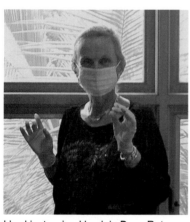

I had just arrived back in Boca Raton. My hair was just starting to grow back. I had to wear the mask to avoid catching the cold George had.

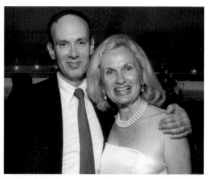

Dr. Robert Press is a friend forever. He told me to go to New York to find out what was wrong with me.

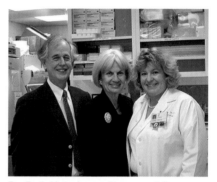

Dr. Ruth Katz, here with me and George, gave us a tour of her research facility at M.D. Anderson Hospital.

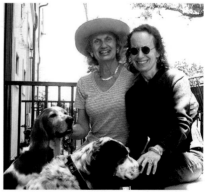

My dear friend, Mary Likosky from Seattle, really lifted my spirits when she visited.

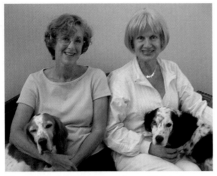

My friend of thirty years, Anna Finkbeiner, traveled from Bermuda to visit me while I was undergoing to treatment.

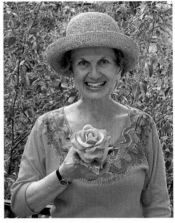

When I could not be around real flowers during my chemotherapy, George brought me this porcelain rose from my Boehm porcelain collection.

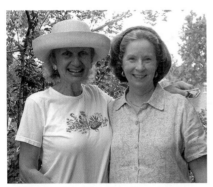

When I first became ill, my friend Evelyn Cathcart took me to the train bound for New York, where I was later diagnosed. Friends are true treasures.

12

People Make a Hospital

The hills are alive and the earth is hummin'
Love is spreadin' over the world!
Put your ear to the ground, you can hear it comin'
Love is spreadin' over the world!

from "Love is Spreading over the World"

July 2002

No matter how advanced the architecture, the food service, or the decor, a hospital can't heal you. It's the human bonds, formed within a hospital, that ultimately lead to healing and to health.

- *Just as you would not want to take a medication without first researching its side effects, you should try not to enter into the care of a hospital or medical center without considering the nature of its staff (sometimes you have no choice, as in a medical emergency).*

I have never seen this truth so forcibly illustrated as when I was at the M.D. Anderson Cancer Center. The exterior beauty of the hospital was eclipsed by the radiance of its staff, and the impact they had on my healing couldn't be measured. The staff at every level—doctors, nurses' aids, and receptionists alike—had the power to make or break my day, and each one became a vital link in the chain I was making to pull myself out of cancer's clutches.

Shea Willis and Willie Mae Singleton must be two of the best phlebotomists ever born. I have "uncooperative veins," which means that my veins test the skill and the mettle of anyone trying to reach them. When it seemed like Shea and Willie Mae had drawn several hundred tubes, I expected even these highly skilled ladies to give up. But as I progressed through my chemotherapy treatments, they only became friendlier and more patient.

The warmth and friendship Shea and Willie Mae radiated—as well as their abundant and genuine care for my health—transformed what could have been a an unpleasant experience into an opportunity to be uplifted. I could easily have let my deflated veins leave me feeling depressed, crestfallen, and drained of life. This would have impacted my ability to sleep soundly, eat well, and stay focused on a successful and complete healing.

Instead, after experiencing their warmth and care, I felt more ready than ever to fight cancer and win. Renewed, refreshed, and energized, I confidently headed for chemotherapy; the next step of my cancer-fighting regime.

This kind of personal care is not just a luxury for a lucky patient in the process of healing: it's a vital part of the healing itself. When we enter into hospital care, our psychological and emotional states change dramatically, and things that may seem trivial to a normal person (like whether the receptionist greets you with a bright smile or ushers you in without a glance) turn into matters of enormous impact on your well-being.

For instance, each time I entered the eighth-floor lymphoma waiting room, Vicki Berera, the receptionist, would greet me with a bright smile saying, "It's great to see you." Sometimes I'd even get a hug.

- *To a patient wrestling with cancer, such a simple exchange becomes profound.*

When your very life is placed into the care of strangers, your mind and emotions fundamentally change. You may have noticed that people who have struggled with sickness tend to recall a handful of random but sharply specific details about their hospital—the way the room looked, whether it was hot or cold, the color of the walls, the dreams they had, and so on. But above all, survivors remember the people who nursed them through their time of struggle and trial, down to their facial features and future plans.

This is because we enter into a heightened state of perception and emotionality when confronted with any major illnesses. As the frailty of the body pushes us closer to the edge of existence, the mind's borders become more flexible, more malleable, and newly diffuse. As a result, we may enter an extreme state of emotional vulnerability and sensitivity.

In this state, the consequences of having an emotionally detached caregiver become vast. An argument between family members in the hallway can have an impact on the suffering patient within, even if the effect is not immediately apparent. The coolness of a practitioner can make a patient in critical condition feel like giving up and eventually contribute to a decision to let go.

On the other hand, the warmth and care of a loving nurse can inspire a patient to resume the fight for life. What a tremendous job! But this caregiver-patient dynamic doesn't occur exclusively between a nurse and a sick person—it's at work talking to doctors, making appointments with receptionists, communicating with other hospital staff, and doing virtually anything else to help you heal. All of these interactions have the power to dampen your spirit, or to energize you to fight. Because of this, the human beings who provide your health care ideally should be selected as carefully as your plan of attack against cancer.

Once you've decided to go with a certain plan of treatment, it's time to ask an equally important question: who will be administering these treatments? With whom will I be interacting on a daily basis because of these treatments?

Often, Erica Banguera, the scheduler at the Cancer Center, would come out of the back office to say hello to me and to some of the other patients. She made us feel special at a time when our feelings were at their most fragile. If you had a problem, Erica would always help. Somehow, she kept all the schedules straight for my myriad of appointments, so that I never felt overwhelmed or confused. "She certainly is organized; I could take a few lessons from her," I had thought to myself more than once.

Erica was poised, intelligent, caring, and gave me plenty of hugs for encouragement. You could call her if there was a conflict in your schedule and she would always cooperate. Though the title "scheduler" sounds cold and impersonal, her very personal qualities made her an important player in my healing. When I left Erica, I felt optimistic, ready to knock cancer out for good.

One morning, I found out that Erica was starting nursing school, and I knew she would be a blessing for every patient she touched. The quality of health care would be even higher today if more people like Erica were manning the decks.

Your Healing Team

Until the day when Erica's caring kind of quality health care has been established everywhere and the relationship between how a patient *feels* and how a patient *fights* is recognized institutionally, it's up to you to make sure that everyone on your healing team adds an uplifting element.

* *No one should make you feel like giving up. After each interaction, ask yourself this question: On a scale of one to ten, how much do I feel like fighting cancer and winning? If you're getting perfect tens every time, you've found someone for your team. Anything significantly lower than that could mean that you need to ask for another person to fill the slot. I did it myself several times.*

Sometimes you don't think you have a choice, but you do. Never be afraid to speak up and ask for a change.

Friendly Faces

The nurses who administered the chemotherapy tended to become the closest to the patients. Gently and kindly administering toxic chemicals can bring two people together in a strange way. Their loving and kind demeanor helped my mind and body understand that chemotherapy was there to help me, not to hurt me. Norma, Bea, Christine, Mary, and many others administered the toxic chemicals in the most sensitive and delicate way imaginable.

- *Many of the nurses were from the Philippines and had the combined qualities of high technical skill and great compassion that could help me heal. Florence Nightingale would have been proud.*

Late one night I visited the M.D. Anderson emergency room because wild shapes were dancing in my eyes. I saw fires of red, blue, and yellow. I couldn't have known at first hand what tripping on LSD was like, but these sensations must have rivaled such an experience. The episode lasted only five or six minutes, but my husband George insisted that I get checked out without delay.

While in the ER I met Dr. Margaret Row. I never saw a busier person, yet somehow she still took the time to say hello, and to find out what was wrong with me. After several hours of tests by a neurologist, I found out that my visual fire dance was probably just an atypical reaction to one of the drugs I was taking and I was free to leave the hospital with clear vision and my mind at ease.

As I was leaving, I saw three M.D. Anderson security guards standing outside the emergency room door. It was well past midnight.

"Would one of you be kind enough to walk me across the street to the parking lot?"

Immediately, a young man in uniform came forward. "I'll be glad to," he said.

I was relieved, and as we were walking around the corner of the building, there was my husband once again, with a smile on his face. "You're out" he said, as if I had just been released from the Bastille.

"That I am," I answered. "Let's go home!"

"God bless you," the young security guard said, as we waved good-bye and thanked him.

"God bless you too," I said. "You made a real difference."

I wasn't lying. These friendly faces and words stick out in my memory like beacons of hope in the midst of what might seem like endless trial and struggle. I know that these positive experiences made a difference in my fight for life. Though the interactions may have lasted only a few moments, these people reminded me that no matter how much discomfort I felt, there was enough love and warmth in the world to make my life worth fighting for. And fight I did!

The young lady attendant in the Marriott parking lot, Anna Martinez, became another friendly face on my road to the cure. I often left the car with her, because it was across the street from M.D. Anderson, and I liked the quarter-mile walk to the cancer center. I always thought, "power walk!"

Dr. Goy instilled in his patients the precept that "exercise is a key to getting healthy." I'd pull my car up and hand Anna the keys.

"How are you today, Mrs. Parker," she'd inquire with a big smile.

"I'm great," I'd reply enthusiastically.

"I love your attitude, you're going to get better," she'd often say.

"I love life," I'd add, and wave good-bye.

- *As a cancer patient, I was more sensitive to everything in my world. Each time I felt a stroke of caring I would just lap it up and add it to my collection of acts that promote healing and strength.*

It's the human warmth and love that adds so much healing to the patient, no matter what's in the bottle or the intravenous line. People can be pumped full of the best treatments in town, but they're not going to do as well as they might if they don't have the will to fight—and fight hard—for their lives.

- *The willpower to fight for your life ultimately comes from emotional sources and needs to be taken very seriously by health care professionals and patients seeking to understand their own healing process.*

Until every health care industry professional understands and respects his or her power to help or to hurt patients, the obligation will rest with the patient to find the right people to administer treatments. I believe it to be as vital a decision as the treatments themselves.

13

God Had a Plan

So many nights I sit by my window
Waiting for someone to sing me his song
So many dreams I kept deep inside me
Alone in the dark but now You've come along...
from "You Light Up My Life"

I couldn't sleep, no matter what I tried. I read a book, did a crossword puzzle, and attempted to iron. That might make anyone tired. Not me. Nothing seemed to work. As I walked into the bathroom, the full moon was beaming through the window. I love the moon. It has special meaning.

All of a sudden, it was clear as a bell. God had a plan. He knew that if he gave me bronchitis or the flu, I'd stay in bed for a few days and then keep pushing, trying to be everything to everyone, paying little attention to myself.

How could he let me know that I needed to change my ways and remember myself? How could he do it without sending me up to heaven and giving me a good lecture? He had to do something serious, which would prompt me to change my life pattern. I had to eat three meals a day. I had to relax, exercise, and take better care of myself.

Reflecting back to the years that I was at the Concord, running to every dining room table I could within the three-hour meal period, gave me pause for thought. The guests ate and I ran. Now, I understand why I suffered from esophageal reflux, hiatal hernia, and indigestion. I ate on the run so I could greet as many of the guests as possible. I was dealing with the tension of running a huge hotel, the squabbles, and jealousies associated with family businesses, and the final curtain (but that's another book). I thought about stress and how many times I had heard our good friend Dr. Paul Rosch, the President of the American Institute of Stress and recognized expert in the field, talk about good stress and bad stress; and how it could affect your health. Perhaps I had too much of the latter.

It became clear that night that sometimes you have to fall farther than you think possible before you can pick yourself up, dust yourself off, and start all over again! It's become one of my favorite phrases. If I could change my lifestyle and begin the journey again, anyone can. Even though cancer had invaded my life, I was willing to do whatever was necessary to give myself the best chance for recovery.

I contemplated where I had been and what, if given the chance to regain my health, I'd do in the future. Where would destiny take me? Would I become a magazine writer? Would I finish my doctorate in philosophy? Would I continue to fight for the rights of the elderly? Would I follow my father's and Dr. Goy's sage advice and write a book about how I survived cancer, from the notes I had kept each day since it all began? All of these ideas drifted into my mind, and thinking about the possibilities gave me something positive to consider.

- *Cancer patients need to look forward to the future because it builds confidence.*

I wondered what kind of impact I was having on my immediate family. Would they see my inner strength and determination to fight and overcome this disease? Would George be up to the task of living through my emotionally tough times while carrying out his business obligations with all the energy he needed? These were just some of the questions that were flashing through my mind.

Always feeling that whatever you put into your children comes back has now been proven over and over again.

One can't demand love; it must be earned. Love does not emerge, fully flowered, in a day; it grows, much like a tree, over the years.

Just ask George, an expert after thirty-seven years of marriage; he could write the book on what love, care, and commitment are all about. Love is catching. It seems to me regrettable that many people restrain and measure their words and actions to such a degree that others don't know how much they are loved.

It was never the case with me. I happen to be a communicator. Everyone I care about knows it. When cancer arrived on my doorstep, the outpouring of love from others was overwhelming, and I opened my heart to receive all I could embrace.

God is wondrous. He told me to slow down and smell the roses. He decided to give me a curable disease, but I'd have to go through all the therapies, needles, drugs, and hell to survive. He never wanted me to forget how precious my life is and the fact that I can be of real help to no one if I am not in good health. He gave me George, my staunchest supporter, and Amy, my beautiful pregnant daughter about to give birth to our second grandchild. He made us "the parents" of McCoy and McKenzie, our loyal English setters. He moved me to Texas, far away from everyone I knew except John and Chrissy. He had me meet Ruth, who leased me her townhouse five minutes from the hospital. God gave us the support of friends and relatives. He encouraged me but also sent me a stern warning. "Sharon, take care of yourself here on this earth if you want to stay..."

Well, I want to stay, and I'll do everything I can to make sure I'm never so wrapped up in everything else that I forget to take care of myself. Thank you, God. I love you.

14

Emergency Room

I am woman, hear me roar
'Cause I've heard it all before
And I know too much to go back and pretend
Nothing's ever gonna keep me down again
from "I Am Woman"

Dr. Andy Zelenetz at Memorial Sloan-Kettering advised me to live as close as possible to the hospital. Side effects, my age, and any unexpected complications were the reason. No matter what decisions a patient makes in regard to an oncologist or a cancer center, whether it be close to home or farther away, a well-equipped emergency room accustomed to handling cancer patients' reactions and complications is a real plus.

* *Once you are a cancer patient, a visit to the emergency room is a good idea. At the very least, you'll know where to park and whom you should see. Learn the ropes.*

* *An important fact to consider is that your oncologist won't be the one who will be waiting for you in the middle of the night, if something goes wrong. The emergency room doctors at M.D. Anderson were used to handling a long list of problems that can come from radiation, chemotherapy, and low blood counts, just to name a few.*

After paying visits to the ER several times in the middle of the night, I realized what good advice Dr. Zelenetz had offered. The ER is often crowded, and when you don't feel well, knowing that it is close by is a real comfort.

Thinking I was progressing according to plan, George left on a business trip while I nursed an aching arm. Perhaps it was a reaction to Neupogen (filgrastim), the white blood cell booster I had taken over the previous three days. "Not to worry," I said to myself, take Tylenol (acetaminophen). Aspirin was not approved because it makes the platelets weaken. Tylenol is allowed only if you have no temperature. God, did I have any blood left?

After an uneventful day, getting a good night's sleep was foremost on my mind. On my way to the bedroom, I stopped by the kitchen for a cold glass of milk and some peanut butter on crackers. I didn't really need to eat before bed, but peanut butter made me feel like a kid again, and that was a great way to end the day.

At 1:30 A.M., I awoke with a start. Gosh, what's happening? I had a sharp pain under my left breast, which radiated around my back.

"Be calm," I told myself aloud, but even after a few minutes, the pain lingered. What else should I do? I couldn't take aspirin, something you might do if you suspected a heart attack. Had I bent or twisted in the wrong way? Nothing came to mind. I decided to walk down to the kitchen on the floor below and drink some club soda. A small burp emerged, but the pain didn't diminish. It was severe, and the thought of something serious happening crossed my mind. To go or not to go to the hospital in the middle of the night, all alone, became the question.

Deciding that there was no choice, but not wanting to disturb anyone else's sleep with a wailing siren, I drove to the ER by myself. The nurse on duty was visibly upset by my decision not to call an ambulance. She informed me that I had risked my life and that of anyone else on the road, as well. Thank goodness, the streets were almost deserted at 2

A.M. Next time I will heed her advice and wake up the neighborhood.

- *Everyone should have an emergency plan and not be afraid to call an ambulance.*

After a thorough exam, the nurse and the doctor on call decided vacuuming a three-story townhouse, moving some furniture earlier in the day, coupled with the peanut-butter-and-cracker binge at 11 P.M. probably weren't my most brilliant choices.

Greatly relieved to find out that my problem was only indigestion, I drove back home slightly embarrassed but oh so pleased with the outcome.

15

We'll Be Friends Forever

Wherever we go
Whatever we do
We're gonna go through it
together...

from "Together"

Any cancer patient will tell you that having a support system is one of the most important parts of the equation in achieving your cure. Family and friends are the first responders, but perfect strangers can become new friends and often fill the void when they learn of your situation. "Merry, Evelyn, and Anna" could have been anyone's friends or relatives.

- *The importance of how they went out of their way and the impact it had on this cancer patient can't be overstated. These three ladies represent everyone who tries to make a cancer patient's journey that much smoother.*

Merry
Merry must have been so named on purpose. Upon the arrival of her flight from Seattle, she took a cab directly to M.D. Anderson. I was thrilled to see her. She was my University of Vermont college sister and has been a true friend for more than forty years. Seeing her grand smile, even if it had to be in the chemotherapy waiting room, lifted my spirits sky high.

She looked so young, yet she was getting her PhD in Greek and Latin studies. "You look like a college kid" I said, tears filling my eyes with joy!

"You look fantastic," she shot back, with a smile that lit up the room like a Christmas tree.

"A little less on my head," I replied, pointing to the thinning hair under my wide-brimmed pink hat. My hair was falling out faster than normal, from the drugs I was being injected with every two weeks.

Brightly colored wide-brimmed hats made me feel better, and I bought several in different colors. We hugged and kissed as she said, "This chemo thing will be fine, and I'm told your hair will grow back after your treatments are over. We'll "chill: like we were in our college dorm and just talk all night."

Once again, the chemo was running late, about three hours this time. At 7 P.M., a lovely Philippine nurse came for me. I explained that I was getting the slow-drip right into my vein. I had no port in my chest. Her name was Norma Urcia, and she had no problem with that fact. This lady would become another new friend who would help me through the chemotherapy until the end.

"I'm getting an ICU nurse to put the needle in," she said brightly; after looking at my tired withered little veins. In just a few minutes, Bea Castillo arrived with a smile. I could sense the kindness and tender touch of this highly skilled Philippine nurse right away. That put me at ease almost immediately. The IV was set on the first try. In five hours we were done; saline, ondansetron (Zofran), dexamethasone (Decadron), and ABVD were swimming around in my body once again.

We ventured home right after the therapy, with Merry in the passenger seat. She couldn't believe I had the strength to drive. It was my way of showing that I was still capable and independent. Chemo #6 was finally over, and I spent the rest of the night on and off the toilet, trying to get all the little poisons out of my system while also drinking a large volume of water. Would all this do the trick and kill the cancer? Only time would tell.

The desire to have fun again without worrying about cancer cells sprouting up somewhere else in my body entered my mind, but only for a moment.

Three days with Merry made me see "springtime." We laughed, cried, hugged, and shared our children's triumphs and concerns. We helped each other and had a wonderful time just being together.

I was feeling much better as I drove her back to the airport, and she was thrilled that she had had such a positive impact on my spirits.

"You'll lick this thing and I'm coming back to Houston," she said without skipping a beat.

I had no doubt that she was right on both counts!

After Merry's departure, I continued to gain confidence by cooking, cleaning, laughing, playing piano, singing, and taking the dogs for an evening drive. When not at home, I could often be found at M.D. Anderson getting my blood tested, receiving Procrit and Neupogen, and trying to be upbeat, positive, and smiling. I felt more secure living very close to the hospital, near the people I trusted. I was making progress and doing as much as I could to achieve my ultimate goal of being a healthy, vibrant woman.

Evelyn

Chemo #7 was right around the corner and I was anxious to get going. Evelyn would join me next, in the heat of the summer. "A great tribute!" I thought to myself, as I looked at the thermometer registering 106°F.

Evelyn arrived at Bush International Airport. It was a sunny day, with the temperature just tipping 96°F. I drove the twenty miles to meet her at 2 P.M. Unfortunately, I made the mistake of getting out of the car to ask a police officer if I were in the right location. It was steaming hot and I didn't notice the step. In a split second, my body landed hard on the concrete.

I developed a habit of blaming anything that went amiss on the chemotherapy. I cut my hand just enough to make it bleed. Knowing the importance of washing my wound right away to avoid an infection, the search for a bottle of water in the car began. Knowing that water was a necessity, I usually had a few extras in the back, but not that day.

Seeing me fall, a police officer came to my rescue. After telling her that I was an M.D. Anderson cancer patient, she brought me a bottle of water right away, so I could wash the bruise. It was a typical Houstonian response. Over and over, people have shown the true meaning of kindness.

Evelyn was very concerned about my hand.

"I told you I could take a taxi," she said considerately.

"Don't be silly. It's Sunday—no traffic. I just did something stupid."

I told her about my silly accident, we were relieved that there was no infection, and the slight injuries disappeared in a few days.

I was hoping everything would go smoothly with my treatments. Already finished with chemo #6, I was looking forward to showing Evelyn how I'd mastered all the techniques. She and her husband Charles had followed my progress from day one.

• *Loyalty, like love, is something rare and priceless. Love is one of the best things about life. Because cancer is emotionally draining, the love and caring that is shown to a patient can't be overestimated.*

It was time for my seventh chemotherapy session. About one hundred people were also waiting to have their blood checked at 8 A.M. I knew that meant a long delay, which had become routine. People had their blood tests either prior to bone marrow aspiration, stem cell collection, transfusion, or chemotherapy. Finally my name was called. Meanwhile, Evelyn watched in awe at the sheer number of patients and the massive scale of M.D. Anderson. Within the hour, we had the results in hand and were off to see Dr. Goy.

Large numbers of people were already in the area marked Lymphoma. The names of these designated cancer treatment areas were no longer scary to me. I'd go in with a purpose and a smile. I showed the doctor a bruise on my hand, a lump on my arm, and some yellow phlegm that I had collected in a plastic bag. They didn't seem to deter him.

"Chemo as usual," he declared with a smile.

"How fortunate I am to have an optimistic doctor like this," I'd say repeatedly to anyone who would listen. His other patients felt the same way I did. We would often discuss his unique abilities while waiting patiently to see him. My schedule said 4 P.M., but when I went to the second floor bed unit, the nurses were running two hours behind. Sixty-three patients were ahead of me. When the nurse on duty asked me if I could come back at 7 P.M., I was quick to oblige, since I lived only five minutes away.

Evelyn and I drove back to the townhouse and made chicken salad, something any two friends spending a few hours together might do. We played the piano, and I taught her some chords. We relaxed in warm baths and exercised while awaiting George's arrival. He was driving from Boca Raton. He arrived close to 6 P.M. and was delighted to find a steak and fried potatoes hot off the grill. He looked wonderful: who would have guessed he had driven the past fourteen hours straight to be with me in time for chemo #7?

It was time to return to M.D. Anderson. We gave each of the dogs a milk-bone, and left the TV on Animal Planet—their favorite station. George went right to bed for a much-needed nap.

When we arrived, the waiting room was still crowded and I knew there was a long night ahead of us. Signing the registration, I gave the receptionist two boxes of gourmet chocolate-chip cookies for the staff to nibble. Most of the nurses didn't take time for a break on very busy nights, and I tried to do my part to help them. It made me feel like I was contributing something in a very small way before my next chemotherapy would begin.

As sometimes happens, chemo #7 was not one to write home about. Evelyn was very concerned because I was crying after it was over but didn't know why. The nurse had accomplished everything and the needle was inserted properly, but something was missing; I felt sick to my stomach and way under par.

"What is wrong?" Evelyn repeated the question.

"I don't know!" I answered between the tears. "I just feel lousy."

It was the following day when I found out that Decadron (dexamethasone), a synthetic corticosteroid had inadvertently been left out of my chemo-cocktail mix of drugs.

* *Decadron is used in chemotherapy; it is an anti- inflammatory drug that reduces the nausea and makes the patient more willing to continue with the regimen.*

Even so, I was able to drive home. Evelyn offered, but I still had to prove to myself and those that cared that I was competent and self-sufficient.

That independence repeatedly helped prove that I could do it even under adverse conditions.

* *Believing in yourself and getting positive feedback for your accomplishments helps to build your confidence.*

By the next morning, I was feeling much better. Evelyn and I talked most of the night as the poisons passed through me and departed by way of the toilet. She could make me laugh, and her bright blue eyes were a sparkling reminder of good things to come. I told her about my Uncle Jack, who was superstitious about saying that things were going great.

"Say 'they're going as well as can be expected'," he'd said to me in a recent phone call. I decided from then on to heed his advice.

Dr. Goy advised me repeatedly to stay focused on the positive aspects of my life. He suggested living as normally as possible and building up my mind and body every day. It was very good advice and reminded me that I could do anything I was asked to do. Moderation was the key.

Anna

Anna Finkbeiner had been a special friend of mine for more than thirty years. In the seventies, her husband Horst managed a famous St. Maarten hotel called Mullet Bay. Nearby, on that tropical Caribbean paradise, George and his dad were building the Concord Hotel on Maho Bay.

I had arrived on this half-French and half-Dutch island, with Amy, aged fifteen months, and little John, just four weeks old. We lived at the edge of the shimmering sea, for six years. My closest neighbor, around the bend, was Anna Finkbeiner, who was raising two little boys and a girl. She was originally from beautiful Bermuda.

There we were on a rather primitive island back in 1968, with five offspring between us. We shared toys, formulas, milk, diapers, and anything else that would make life easier. We never lost touch, and even though our paths went in different directions, we have always been there for one another.

Anna was shocked when I told her what was happening to me.

"I'll be there, girl," she said, during a call from Bermuda.

I told her that Merry, Evelyn, and my sister Ellen had already come to see me. I wanted her to wait until I was finished with chemo so we could go out and play, as we used to with the children. I told her about the fabulous Houston Zoo, and we decided that we would definitely spend a day, "talking to the animals."

When Dr. Goy mapped out the chemotherapy schedule, I realized that I'd need to stay in Houston for a few weeks to recover. Then the doctors would scan my body again to make sure the cancer was dead and buried. That would be the perfect time for Anna to arrive.

As before with Merry and Evelyn, we felt like young women, laughing and crying and discussing green tea and Tai Chi. Anna was insisting I dance more and worry less.

I told her that I chose to stay away from anyone with serious or unusual infections. A call to the doctor is always advisable when you are not sure. I became vigilant about handwashing. I tried to do everything I could to stay healthy. I didn't consume sushi or raw fruits and vegetables. Common sense is a must.

It was an education for both of us as we visited the different floors of M.D. Anderson. Anna had never seen so many people with cancer, but she confided to me that she was concerned about a suspicious lump on her breast.

We had a marvelous time eating health-consciously. We enjoyed romaine lettuce, poached salmon with dill, lots of grains, and so on. When we hugged each other as she was departing, she promised to get that breast checked again.

Sure enough, it turned out to be a malignant tumor. Now, I am helping her get through courses of chemotherapy and radiation. She is a real trooper, and in my heart, I know that she too will get well.

- *No one ever knows when cancer may strike, but all of us need to be alert. Cancer is an unpleasant fact of life. It can strike anyone at any time but it does not have to be the end.*

16

The ABCs of Lymphoma

In the little red school house
With my book and slate
In the little red school house
I was always late
from "In the Little Red School House"

May 24, 2002

The mind works in strange ways. It's what decides when "enough is enough" or when it is time to absorb something new. All of us can relate to that. Just think back to high school, when you were conjugating French verbs while trying, at the same time, to memorize the theorems in geometry! Personally, I remember thinking "What do I need geometry for? I'm not going to be an architect!" How we look at new information and whether we choose to absorb it has to do in part with whether we want the knowledge at all.

Cancer patients are no different from anyone else. There are those who are immediately curious about what has invaded their bodies and who therefore try to learn everything they can. And then there are others who want to know as little as possible, in the hope that their illness will disappear one day. Finally, there are those who want to know but can't cope with one more scintilla of information or who are just not ready to personalize the scary material that is presented. I fell into this latter group.

In looking back, I remember the day I walked into the cancer library at the Marriott by myself and became overwhelmed glancing through all of the booklets and videos regarding cancer statistics and the chances of survival. I wasn't

100

ready for any of it. The timing wasn't right. But then things changed. My curiosity came back, along with a capacity to absorb new information.

Moving in a positive direction and ready to forge ahead and get educated suddenly became of interest to me. It was a fact of life that I had cancer, and I had nothing to lose by learning. It didn't take long for my curiosity to blossom. I yearned to know what Hodgkin's disease really was and how it related to lymphoma. What I've come to realize is that timing is everything.

A simple soft-covered medical guide from the local Barnes and Noble was my first purchase. It was not only about my disease but included data on other cancers as well. It made me realize that plenty of people are stricken with cancer. I was certainly not alone in the world and I would continue my fight to get better.

Sometimes the facts became more than I could absorb; they became unsettling. Eventually I understood that my mind can concentrate on only one thing at a time. Therefore, when I felt overwhelmed, I'd stop and do anything that made me smile, like watching a comedy on television or playing the piano.

- *If your cup becomes too full, change your focus until you're ready to learn a little more. It is remarkable how quickly your mind adapts and emotions rebound.*

Of course for me, learning about the lymphoid system had never been a priority. The idea that thin vessels branch into all parts of the body carrying a watery, clear liquid called lymph seemed foreign to me. I didn't remember learning about it in Biology 101.

Reading further, I found that lymphocytes and other white blood cells circulate throughout the system and comprise a major component of the defense team that fights infection. In addition, all along the system are tiny bean-shaped nodes, which you can sometimes feel in the underarm area or along the neck. These lymph nodes make and store a number of the infection-fighting cells; I never realized that my tonsils, spleen, and thymus gland were all part of this system—it had never mattered before.

A healthy body is full of normal lymphocytes (cells of the immune system). Viruses, ionizing radiation, chemicals, or other factors can damage them, causing mutations to occur within one or several of the genes controlling cell growth, division, or recycling.

These now abnormal cells can become, over time, malignant tumors called Hodgkin's or non-Hodgkin's lymphomas, which are cancers of the immune system.

One of the major differences between the two lymphoma types is that Hodgkin's lymphoma spreads in a contiguous manner, from node to adjoining node, while non-Hodgkin's lymphoma tends to spread more rapidly and systemically through the bloodstream.

Hodgkin's disease was described in 1832 by Thomas Hodgkin, a London physician.

Dr. Crawford had mentioned early on at NYU, that Hodgkin's lymphoma was easier to cure than the non-Hodgkin's type.

Malignant tumors contain cells that multiply uncontrollably and invade surrounding tissue. Our normal cells are then crowded out by these rebels and are unable to function properly. If left untreated, affected organs are rendered unable to perform their life-sustaining functions.

The kind of lymphoma that chose to invade my body had cells that looked abnormal under high-magnification microscopy. They're called Reed-Sternberg cells, named for their discoverers and believed to be a class of malignant lymphocytes. When my biopsy was studied at the NYU Medical Center, Dr. Crawford said he was very surprised to see those very distinctive cells glaring back at him.

Some symptoms that might lead to a diagnosis of Hodgkin's disease include *night sweats, weight loss, itching, and fatigue.* These warning signs seemed strange to me because we live in a hot, muggy climate and I love to sleep un-

102

der all of my northern covers. Sweating is considered normal in Florida for almost everyone, including a fifty-eight-year-old postmenopausal woman.

Talking about weight loss, many of us women are on a perpetual diet, trying to stay between a size 8 and a 10. Fats don't agree with me anyway, so I thought weight loss was a good omen. Bugs and humans live side by side in the Sunshine State and bites are a common occurrence. I thought that an itch meant that some little critter was hungry and just had lunch on me. Never did I think it could mean cancer. Fatigue? I was always exhausted but kept pushing myself. Working hard every day was the norm for me. I thought everyone else felt tired as well. Perhaps if I had known the warning signs earlier, I would have been more aware of what my body might be trying to tell me.

According to the American Cancer Society, lymphoma affects approximately 70,000 people annually, and the number is growing. Of those, eight thousand will be diagnosed with Hodgkin's disease. The National Cancer Institute says that thyroid cancer, in different forms, strikes nearly 24,000 people annually. It was hard for me to believe that two cancers, simultaneously, were doing their best to destroy me. Thank God they were recognized early, and I hoped that I would be able to annihilate them, before they could obliterate me!

The American Cancer Society's Seven Warning Signs

Change in bowel or bladder habits

A sore, that does not heal

Unusual bleeding/discharge

Thickening/lump in breast or elsewhere

Indigestion/difficulty in swallowing

Obvious change in warts or mole

Nagging cough/hoarseness

17

To Radiate or Not to Radiate, That Is the Question

The choice of whether to receive radiation is not often an option for people with cancer. When the chemotherapy was nearing its end, the topic once again surfaced.

In many instances, chemotherapy and subsequent radiation are used to make certain that all of the malignant cells are truly dead.

Whether this is necessary in every instance is a question that oncologists see differently. Most of us are aware that too much radiation is not a good thing, but sometimes there is no viable alternative. Therefore these rays are still considered mainstream for both diagnostic testing as well as the destruction of cancer cells.

For some of us however, there may be a choice. If it weren't for the expertise and concern of my doctors, I might never have known.

Toward the beginning, my rude awakening to the fact that I might indeed have a shortened life span pushed me to gather all the information I could on ABVD chemotherapy as well as on the possible side effects of radiation therapy.

Dr. Goy had told me from the beginning that I might need it, but he had a wait-and-see attitude, depending on my body's response to chemotherapy.

When I found out that Hodgkin's disease had invaded my upper chest through the lymphatic system, I saw hematologist oncologist, Kenneth Hymes at NYU Medical Center. He was the skilled physician who told me, early on, that my bone marrow looked healthy. That information was critical, because it enabled him to evaluate the extent of the disease. In my case, the cancer cells were still in the lymph nodes and had not spread systemically.

Dr. Hymes then wrote a report asserting that radiation might not be in my best interest because I didn't have a bulky tumor, which typically requires a combination of chemotherapy and radiation.

Instead, the Hodgkin's disease had spread all across my upper body above the diaphragm. This would have required an extensive field of radiation, which would have put me at risk for other cancers. Always grateful for Dr. Hymes' early report, I shared it with Dr. Goy, whom I knew was receptive to hearing the ideas of others in the field.

Because I had been astute enough to ask for copies of every report and each test, I had a lot of information to process. Compiling a notebook was one of my most important accomplishments, because these documents contained everything the doctors had established in my particular case.

- *I urge you to compile a notebook. The information in it could prove to be invaluable.*

Now there was something else to add to the equation: In some cases, thyroid cancer may be the result of too much radiation. What I found is that there are differing opinions on just how much is too much.

I hadn't been in a radioactive fallout zone that I knew of and certainly had not been in Chernobyl, in 1986, when the world's worst nuclear reactor accident occurred. So, how could I have been overradiated?

Perhaps I had had too many x-rays during my life. Trying to remember all of them was impossible. In addition, many dental visits required x-rays, and no one ever covered my thyroid gland, which is located at the base of the neck.

The big heavy lead apron was put on, but that only went to the extreme base of my neck. We all need to be aware that the dentist leaves us alone during the x-ray, as do all x-ray technicians. Be smart and ask for protection of your neck area as well. The last thing we need is another cancer popping up.

Since radiation is cumulative and exactly how many rads you receive is critical, it is important for all of us to weigh the importance and frequency of the radiation we receive.

• *Not being doctors, we need guidance and recommendations from those who know more than we do. Ask the questions that are relevant to your own case. "Knowledge is power," and cancer patients need as much of that as possible.*

The day finally arrived for a conference with the radiation oncologist at M.D. Anderson. He explained that this therapy has been used for fifty years.

"What is the downside?" I heard myself ask. George, right beside me, was a bit surprised at the question. But I had done my homework.

When the radiation oncologist was finished listing the possible side effects, he told us of the pluses and minuses. To be honest, I wasn't convinced that radiation treatments were in my best interest, especially because of the thyroid cancer in my neck.

After discussing the recommendation with Dr. Goy and Dr. Sherman, I decided to wait. Radiation could be given down the road if necessary. But if it turned out that I didn't need it, why expose myself to it? Dr Sherman was vigilant in watching my blood counts in regard to the thyroid cancer from the moment of my initial diagnosis, while I continued taking the synthetic thyroid hormone. He also had me repeat the sonograms every twelve weeks and finally every six months to look for any changes. Nothing of significance had appeared after the initial minute focus of thyroid cancer. Had it been killed by the ABVD chemotherapy? I was very optimistic and hopeful but at the same time realistic and ready to move forward if any symptoms, however slight, should appear.

It all sounded reasonable to us. We had a plan, and getting stronger each day would be my number-one priority for now.

18

Why E-Mail?

Love letters straight from your heart
Keep us so near while apart
I'm not alone in the night
When I can have all the love you write

from "Love Letters"

If the feeling of isolation and loneliness creeps into your mind while undergoing chemotherapy, join the crowd. Many of us experience negative feelings while conquering cancer.

Try to remember that we are alive and that the chosen therapy is killing those cancer cells that made our bodies home. To build my spirit and boost my morale, I took a proactive stance. When I became aware that my white blood cell count had dropped, I was careful not to catch an infection. Unpeeled fruits, vegetables, or raw foods such as sushi were off my menu. Dr. Goy had warned me to "live my life" and use common sense, but be concerned about a low white count.

- *Cancer patients sometimes need their own "security blankets." I know I did, especially on those days when my white counts dropped precipitously, not knowing if I was at risk of catching an infection that might prevent me from having more chemotherapy. I decided to wear a surgical face mask if I needed to be around people whose health status was questionable. It gave me confidence at those times to go about my business in my usual way, and since others were wearing masks as well, it made no difference. Ask your oncologist if you have any questions.*

• *Taking part in activities that are perceived as constructive has proven to be beneficial for anyone but especially for cancer patients.*

• *"Alone time" should be a positive experience, and it often is when you feel you've accomplished something. Even perfectly healthy people spend time by themselves. It is because cancer patients are going through physical and emotional changes that being alone can become a negative experience. The idea is to reverse that feeling and make lemonade out of the lemons we are handed.*

Many times, I suggested to George that he go out. I knew that, like all caregivers, he needed time to regenerate, regroup, and renew his spirit. Then he would come back refreshed.

While he was gone or late at night, if I sometimes couldn't sleep, I'd go to my new friend, the Internet. Even though I was far from an expert, I learned to communicate my thoughts and share ideas.

This became one of my most positive experiences and some people actually saved my thoughts for future reference.

Whenever I'd get the urge to write an e-mail, I'd sit down and convey any new information I had learned from the doctor, nurses, or dietitian at the cancer clinic. The emotions and feelings I was experiencing became a part of the Internet and represented my connection to our great big world.

The e-mails helped me remember that my interpersonal activities were limited. My connection to the people who mattered most was not. Still, I had the ability to be a contributing member of society and perhaps one or two of the things that I conveyed would be helpful to someone else.

- *Sharing such personal information may seem difficult for some of us, but we are all one big family when it comes to cancer, and anything that we can do to help each other has to be worthwhile.*

- *Perhaps the best part is the feeling of fulfillment you'll have after you send your e-mails out. The replies you receive will overwhelm you with their love, concern, and thanks for information that just may save someone else's' life.*

Subject: Chemo cocktail #101
Date: 5/18/2002 11:39:07 A.M. Eastern Daylight Time
From: SLPGNP
To: Sharon's Med

My Dear Friends and family,

I have finally mastered the art of how to e-mail to more than one person at the same time like you all know how to do.

We are celebrating my first CHEMO COCKTAIL, and so far so good. I have to admit that I had taken a $39 antinausea pill, and considering my body is worth a total of $2.98 tops, it's seems like quite an outrage.

I must be blessed to have Hodgkin's stage 2A lymphoma, because they think they know how to beat it. My doctor is "charmant, charmant," from France. Many people on the faculty are from other countries and in fact, the pathologist, named Ruth Rheingold Katz, is from Johannesburg and has been an absolute angel to me. M.D. Anderson is huge. I don't know how they keep track of all the people, but they certainly do!

I am very blessed that I found this early. If you don't feel right, keep asking those questions until you get the correct answer. A chest x-ray saved my life and for any of you who have put that off: don't, especially if you have a dry, allergic type cough. Remember in Charleston, in the beginning of April, I was told I was suffering from allergies and given a prescription for Allegra. This happens all too often.

I have 11 more treatments to go, so I am taking one day at a time. Every day may not be as good as this, but I have much to be thankful for.

Houston and John go together. He and Chrissy have been my angels. Amy, Aaron, and Amanda are in production for our latest grandchild. I am so glad I went to Jamesville to see them six weeks ago. Amanda is scrumptious.

To all my friends who have known about this from the inception and have helped me get to where I am, I will never forget your kindness, love, and friendship. This can be conquered. You just have to live through it.

George has been simply fantastic and rose mightily to the occasion. He has boosted my spirits and we are looking forward to a great future.

Love, Sharon

Subject: Amy's Birthday
Date: 5/29/2002 9:48:52 A.M. Eastern Daylight Time
From: SLPGNP
To: Sharon's med

Dear Family, Friends, and Loved Ones,

I hope you are all having a good day. It's especially meaningful to me because today is Amy's birthday. I can't believe that she is thirty-five. That must make me about 50—only kidding. I am thrilled to be on this earth to celebrate with my daughter, even if I am in Houston. Happy Birthday to you, Amy.

Friday I have my Chemo 202. I look at each one as a graduate school seminar, lasting about five hours. I look at it not with fear but with great anticipation, knowing that these drugs are what I need to eradicate cancer from my system.

I don't always feel well because the side effects are un-settling, but as long as they go away, I will just deal with them one at a time. It's scary when you get strange pains in your jaw or extremities.

I am thrilled to have John and Chrissy nearby who have been a fabulous family to have close at hand. They would be here in a second if I need them. I go to their house when-ever I feel great. John made me a beautiful steak and baked potato on Memorial Day, and I have felt better ever since.

George has done a yeoman's job in getting our lives, bills, insurance, etc. in order. Who knew when I left Charleston that day that I'd end up with cancer and in Houston, Texas? "One never knows, does one," as they say. Mc-Coy, McKenzie and their dad are on the way to the "Lone Star State" as we speak. Texas is still booming. Thank God. Bless you all, and thanks for caring.

Love, Sharon

Subject: Chemo 202
Date: 6/7/2002 11:39:07 A.M. Eastern Daylight Time
From: SLPGNP
To: Sharon's Med

Hi,

Here is the latest update on your favorite M.D. Ander-son patient. I must really love you a lot, because I just fin-ished writing to you about all the latest goings on with Chemo 202 last Friday, and just as I was writing the closing, AOL said "good-bye." Oh, I hate that. So here is my second attempt. I am writing this in Microsoft Word and saving it forever. Then I will attach it over to you somehow, I hope.

Chemo cocktail #202 is my graduate school seminar; at least that's what I've gotten my brain to think. I go in with a very positive attitude knowing I will be poked, prodded, and analyzed for the day. I'm almost like the monkey in the research class. I generously gave myself an "A" for attitude, perseverance, and follow-through.

George came home with me only to watch me stay up most of the night, drink bottled water, and make frequent trips to the bathroom. I am not alarmed at the color that leaves my body because one of the drugs is a lovely shade of pink.

My lips and mouth tend to dry up like a wrinkled prune and bottled water is the answer. Pure lanolin on my lips makes them feel better. I've also learned that lip and mouth sores can send you into despair because you can't put anything in your mouth. Ah, but they have a pill for that too and I am feeling a whole lot better than I did yesterday.

So, what is the result of all of this? Onward and forward, it is a learning experience every day. I know I will get through it as I collect my hair that is now leaving my head; I'll make a gorgeous pillow, in the future as a souvenir of my experience. Some people just cut it off or shave their heads. Not me, I am a collector and love beautiful things. I can make something out of nothing and so I will with my locks. You will see it will be a work of art. I hope you are healthy happy and celebrating life as I am.

I love you,
Sharon

_____

Subject: Happy Father's Day
Date: 6/16/2002 11:54:56 P.M. Eastern Daylight Time
From: SLPGNP
To: Sharon's Med

Happy Father's Day. We all have one or had one, so greetings are in order. I often think about my own dad Mike Strauss, who at ninety is still covering the races at Saratoga for the *Palm Beach Daily News*.

I had started the weekend feeling awful but I have ended it with strength and determination to conquer this. There are mountains and valleys in this cure.

This weekend I was climbing Everest and I wasn't sure I was going to make it. I wasn't able to get my chemo cocktail on schedule because my blood count was not high enough. So, I was given two shots of "hell" that would improve the counts. What I didn't know was that I could have a reaction as the Neupogen and Procrit entered all my departments, like my musculo- skeletal system. I thought my body was in a revolt and pain was everywhere.

I am glad to report that as it came, it went. Thank God for Tylenol, which is the only pain medication I can take. I feel fine again and I surely hope that you do too. John made a wonderful Father's Day celebration and even the dogs participated with giant milk bones. I feel very blessed to have celebrated yet another holiday.

I wish I were with you to celebrate together, but we shall have many more wondrous days in the future. You are missed and I thank you for all your kind thoughts, good wishes, and prayers.

Love, Sharon

Subject: Put a smile on your face
Date: 6/26/2002 7:05:59 A.M. Eastern Daylight Time
From: SLPGNP
To: Sharon's Med

Dear loved ones,

I thought I'd let you know that I am moving right along, reaching for the stars and loving the moon. I am very happy and blessed because these past four days I had my children and scrumptious Amanda Grace out here in Houston. Nothing can put a smile on your own face quicker than a child's delight in seeing you! I sang to her most of the time. She is a little dickens and even though her daddy was not able to come, he heard about her accomplishments via the phone. I think she may become a vet. She had three dogs to play with— McCoy, McKenzie, and Lynsie, John's English setter.

John and Chrissy were a wonderful uncle and auntie and Amanda Grace was definitely in control. Amy is expecting our second grandchild in August and is a most beautiful pregnant lady. Small things give you great pleasure when you are not feeling your best—watching Chrissy in the pool with Amanda, watching Amy do Itsy Bitsy Spider with such warmth and seeing the huge smiles on Amanda's face makes the hard times vanish. Hearing her shout "Uncle, Uncle," as she eagerly awaits John's arrival and hugs, lots of hugs.

Grandpa George got his share of laughter too when he arrived for dinner and he brought Amanda an inflatable pool, which is a definite must in Houston's heat. Even the dogs took a dip. Tomorrow morning they leave us with wonderful memories as they head back to New York. I go get some blood taken to see how my counts are doing, and hopefully all will be right with the world.

I love you.
Sharon

Subject: Learning to live with cancer
Date: 7/2/2002 11:04:33 A.M. Eastern Daylight Time
From: SLPGNP
To: Sharon's Med

Hi Loved Ones,

"Cancer calling." It doesn't sound so awful to me anymore. It's just like anything else. You learn to adjust. I am doing fine right now. I visited my handsome French doctor yesterday, and he seems very pleased. I am the only chemo cocktail—make mine a martini—that is gaining weight and growing fingernails. The regular route is to lose them, and I mean quickly.

I am trying to eat healthy, but on occasion, I indulge. Take yesterday, on the way to the hospital I just happened to stop and get half a corned beef sandwich to go with a root beer to boot; it felt great to go off my regular routine and Dr. Goy said it was all OK. I'm allowed to splurge once in awhile.

I am soon going over to M.D. Anderson for my chemo cocktail #4. Amy tells me to do them in threes, and then it won't seem like so many. Good thinking. I just hope and pray for a good nurse who is a great vein finder. That can make all the difference. Have faith, hope, and charity, and think of me.

Love,
Sharon

Subject: (no subject)
Date: 7/6/2002 1:28:21 A.M. Eastern Daylight Time
From: SLPGNP
To: Sharon's Med

Dear Loved Ones,

It has taken me a few days after chemo 4 to write and tell you how delightful it was, because this one was not a piece of chocolate cake. In fact, you know how I love chocolate, but this was pistachio at best. I felt green when I staggered out of the hospital's 10th floor wing. You never know where they are going to send you to get this mustard gas injected into you, and the problem was it was preholiday. Hurry, hurry get the stuff in was the attitude, and that was the problem. PAIN and more pain. My poor veins had a tantrum, but I am much better now and thrilled that I lived to see fireworks from my window on July 4th. I wish we were dancing and singing. I wish that no one else had to go through this. I will do it once for all those I love and who love me. You are in my heart.

Love, Sharon

Subject: Chemo Cocktail #5
Date: 7/14/2002— 10:37:00 P.M. Eastern Daylight Time
From: SLPGNP

To: Sharon's Med

Blast off for Chemo cocktail 5. Estimated time 4:30 P.M. tomorrow. I am waiting with great anticipation and will have blood drawn in the morning to make sure the white count is satisfactory. If it is, Dr. Goy will issue the orders, and I will begin the five or six hour plan.

I have learned a wonderful secret this week. Neupogen and Procrit can be put in your thigh—which seems to hurt a lot less than in your arm—to raise your blood counts, which are lowered from all the drugs. It hurts a lot less, and for that I am so thankful.

I heard from so many friends, children, and loved ones this week. I am not the only patient. Evelyn's daughter, Betsey Cathcart's chocolate lab has also been suffering terribly, but seems to be pulling through with Lyme disease as we speak. She was so good to me when I was in New York. I'll never forget her caring kindness.

Also, big news, Amy is getting ready for her next child to be born. Aaron took Amanda Grace on a business trip to Chicago. I hope Amy is getting a much-needed rest, although I know how much she misses my scrumptious grandchild. Having them out here did wonders for me. I can't wait for my next grandchild who will arrive sometime around August 11th.

John and Chrissy are on a much-deserved vacation. I am thrilled that they will have some free time together.

I am playing the piano every day and find it very relaxing. I am also riding my exercise bike, at least three miles per day, per the doctor's orders, to keep strong.

I am trying so hard to stay healthy and do everything right. I pray for my friends John Romero and Sandy Shwartz in Tuxedo. These weird diseases have just got to go. I love Dirk Salz and Judy's e-mails, and of course Evelyn and Charles' constant wishes. Uncle Jack, Aunt Mame, Barbara,

Sandy, Stephanie, Arnold and all of you who keep my spirits soaring, I thank you. I can't wait until this is over and we can celebrate another victory in life.

Zosia, Serene, Glovina stay healthy. My dear friends that is what really matters. Alexa I love you and all your efforts. George I could not do this without your support and love. Here is to tomorrow. Bless you all.

Love,
Sharon

Subject: (no subject)
Date: 7/28/2002 11:12:09 P.M. Eastern Daylight Time
From: SLPGNP
To: Sharon's Med

Dear Loved Ones,

Tomorrow I celebrate my sixth chemo cocktail. Although I only take one day at a time, so far so good. I feel like the drugs have hit their target, and if the nurses can find a ready and willing vein, I will be ready for them. I think God had a plan for me. He was kind enough to give me a disease that is easier to treat, but I know I need to take better care of me. Every day doctors are coming up with theories about why we get these diseases. I am doing as much as is comfortable, including riding my bike, playing the piano, cooking, and eating. I am grateful to be here and will be elated when this is over. I hope you are well and taking good care of yourself. I can't tell you how much I appreciate your support and love.

Sharon

Subject: Six More To Go
Date: 8/2/2002 10:12:14 P.M. Eastern Daylight Time
From: SLPGNP
To: Sharon's Med

It's not always easy. I am so happy I have reached August. I have finished six chemo cocktails. No matter how I look at it, that means six more. At least that is a lot less than twelve. I have found wonderful nurses, and I only hope they will be mine for the duration.

I have learned that in life there are never any certainties—just hopes and dreams. This week was more exhausting, and I slept through too many hours. It is because chemo is cumulative, and the side effects can be different with each go around. Still, I am able to get up, smile, whirlpool, play the piano, write, ride my bike, cook, clean a bit and enjoy the dogs.

Once again, George has been a rock. I have learned that there are people who don't know what to say; so they say nothing, hoping the disease won't touch them. Cancer is strange. I can think of many reasons why I probably was a good candidate. I am just gratified that perhaps I will mend "good as new." I'd not change the kind of person I am and would outstretch my hand many times again.

George has left on a business trip, so I am in charge. John is a very busy man, but I always know that he and Chrissy are there for me. Amy will be blessing us soon with our latest grandchild. If only we could have peace and love in our world, we would all be much better off.

Love and so many thanks to you, who have really cared.
Sharon

Subject: Chemo Cocktail #7
Date: 8/11/2002 10:34:22 P.M. Eastern Daylight Time
From: SLPGNP
To: Sharon's Med

"Would you prefer a whiskey sour or a gin and tonic? Oh, on this rather warm August day, I'll have an AVBD." That's the name of the concoction I shall be savoring, God willing, tomorrow. First, they'll check my blood to make sure I still have some. Then the good doctor pokes, prods and asks questions. If I pass the test, "I'll go straight to go," and by the end of the day, I'll be home counting my friends, relatives, and blessings.

Our newest blessing and latest news is Andrea Claire, the sister of Amanda Grace! We are also blessed, because Amy is doing well. Aaron is a great father, and Grandparents Sue and Norman Sumida are in Jamesville, New York, to assist in the entire goings on with the new baby.

George is in Pensacola on his way here, after a business trip. The best part of the day was picking up Evelyn Cathcart, who came to cheer me on. Evelyn put me on the train in Charleston, when I knew I had better get to New York! She's been with me in mind and spirit all the way. Need I say more? I am thrilled she is here, and I will show her what I go through to get better, of which I am trying my very hardest. So, if you can, think of me tomorrow and hopefully the nurses will not cause too much pain.

Love, Sharon

Subject: Chemo Cocktail #7
Date: 8/16/2002 12:51:35 P.M. Eastern Daylight Time
From: SLPGNP
To: Sharon's Med

Just when you think everything is going well, your veins collapse and the medicine tastes awful. In fact, chemo cocktail 7 is one I'd like to forget except for the fact that Evelyn Cathcart was there to hold my hand and George, Mc-

Coy, and McKenzie treated me with great tenderness. It is now Thursday and I am beginning to feel like myself again, especially after a consult with Dr. Goy, who came to the conclusion that Decadron, a steroid that makes tolerating chemo much easier, had been inadvertently omitted.

I am thrilled Evelyn was here because it did ease the pain and suffering. Tonight, George went to a great deli and brought me a corned beef on rye. Things must be getting better. He also took a picture of Evelyn and me on the back terrace, which I am sharing with you.

Love, Sharon

Subject: (no subject)
Date: 8/22/2002 5:24:40 P.M. Eastern Daylight Time
From: SLPGNP
To: Cathlit

Dear Evelyn,

Oh where does the time go? This was a unique week, as I get ready for chemo #8. I now know what it must be like on LSD. There I was in bed reading a book after having received a Procrit shot on Monday. All of a sudden, red, blue, and yellow flashing lights went parading by my eyes. It lasted seven minutes and was pretty scary. I went to the emergency room and a neurologist was called in. Seven hours later, at almost 2 A.M., I was released. It sort of messed up my week. They think I had a reaction to one of the drugs.

I am so glad you are not here now because it is 105°F with the humidity factor. I love our picture and the beautiful frame. I hope all of the tests will be done after the next chemo to prove that the cancer is gone. That will be a big relief. Sometimes I just dream about being fine and strolling down the avenue. Worth Avenue sounds great to me. We will have a Florida reunion for sure.

Lots of love,
Sharon

Subject: Chemo #8
Date: 8/28/2002 5:37:57 AM Eastern Daylight Time
From: SLPGNP
To: Sharon's Med

Dear Loved Ones,

Chemo 8 is over and that means only four more to go. It is 4:12 A.M. There goes the biological clock. Chemo changes anything that you take as normal and turns it upside down.

This time the orders for Decadron were loud and clear and that made the overall reaction better. I thought I was having it all at 3 P.M. but it didn't start until almost 9 P.M. Getting a patient nurse and an expert to find your vein is worth the wait.

This week I will begin the tests on my entire body to see if all of this has worked. I think it has. I can sing like I used to. My chest feels clear. I still have strong fingernails and some hair. With a hat on only we know. My spirits are high most of the time, especially when I think about everything else, like my fantastic friends and family.

Everyone going through this needs a support system and I feel truly blessed. You have been wonderful to me and I can't wait to see you. John and Chrissy live the closest and it has been a real blessing. Amy and Aaron produced a beautiful baby, Andrea Claire, and I now have great pictures.

It was 111 degrees on my car thermometer the other day. I just waited for it to cool off. John cooked a banquet on Sunday. George bought me a microphone for the piano so I can sing. Exercise every day, drink water, and stay healthy.

Much Love, Sharon

PS. The results are in and there is no evidence of cancer on all of these tests. This is the news every cancer patient dreams of. Perhaps, I am driven like a steam roller to flatten the cells like a pancake—killing them and getting my mind and body into the best shape it has ever been is my ultimate goal.

Subject: America the beautiful
Date: 9/6/2002 10:39:41 P.M. Eastern Daylight Time
From: SLPGNP
To: Sharon's Med

Dear Loved Ones,

As I look forward to Chemo #9 on September 9th, I reflect on yesterday, one of the more complicated, emotional days of my life. I arrived at the hospital at 7:30 for the beginning of the exploration of my body to see if the cancer is anywhere present.

I don't know the answer yet, after having a barium enema, barium swallows, radioactive material, iodine, and assorted other needles jabbed into me. I held it all together until I was told that another intravenous would be necessary and painful.

I looked at the nurse telling me this and said, "I think I need a different nurse."

Unbelievably, an angel appeared who was so gentle; and she didn't hurt, which gave me the strength to have the barium enema, which is no fun.

When I was swallowing my second glass of barium, for the stomach and pelvic scans, I walked through the hospital connector to the nearby Marriott and pretended I was having another banana daiquiri. I sat in the glass-enclosed walkway and looked out the window directly to a new University of Texas Medical Center building with an American flag waving high in the sky. Magnolia trees were looking back at me, and I knew that God was right above the flag.

"I asked him to take this cancer and send it to a planet with no people on it." I hope he heard my message.

You have been so supportive and wonderful to me. I can't tell you how much it has meant. Only two women, per hundred thousand, of my specific age had this disease last year, according to the American Cancer Institute, yet thousands get Hodgkin's and non-Hodgkin's lymphoma. Now that is pretty amazing.

I love you,
Sharon

Subject: Super Mom
Date: 9/16/2002 11:44:22 P.M. Eastern Daylight Time
From: SLPGNP
To: Sharon's Med

Dear Loved Ones,

I know I have not written on my Sharon's med line recently. I have finished chemo cocktail #9 and it went well.

Tragically, my 86-year-old mom, my supermom, was diagnosed up in Danby, Vermont, with pancreatic cancer after having flu-like symptoms for a relatively short time. Since my mom rarely complained about health issues and had never spent any time in a hospital in many years, no one would have guessed that this newly found cancer had already spread into other parts of her body.

George had a very tough time telling me, because he knew how hard I would take it. Since my mother and I had such a loving and solid relationship and there were no unresolved issues between us, my doctor advised that it would not be a good idea for me to fly to Vermont, because of my low blood counts and the higher risk of infection. Dr. Goy left the ultimate choice up to me.

George, John, and Amy along with Amanda Grace and Andrea Claire went with all of their love, compassion, and caring to Danby. John took a video to my mom's bed from me expressing how I feel and how I am with her in spirit and heart. I also sent a tape for my dad of three songs that I sang and pictures so they could see how I was progressing each day.

I spoke to my mom on the phone and to my dad, who assured me that he wanted me to stay in Texas and get rid of the cancer. I was very grateful to hear him. If I could have given my mom a lung, kidney, or anything else there would have been no question what I would have done, but I know that the greatest legacy I can give her is to get well and beat this Hodgkin's disease and thyroid cancer.

She is resting peacefully in Manchester in a nursing home filled with antiques, and she has around-the-clock care. I am greatly relieved that day and night, she will not suffer, and if I am lucky, I will get to see her once more. If not, heaven is the next choice, and my mother will be the queen.

Today a piece of tooth was glued back on the left side of my mouth after the buckle broke. It was hilarious. Dr. Elizabeth Hunsaker, a superb and creative Houston dentist, thought it best that I not bleed at this time, so she came up with an alternative way to keep my mouth intact until all the chemotherapy is over. I wonder if being left-handed has anything to do with eating on the left side? Perhaps I'll ask her next time. Now, I'll have to remember to eat on the right side—or it will be oatmeal and scrambled eggs for the next six weeks. Peace and good health to you my dear ones. You have been my rock.

Love, Sharon

Subject: Chemo Cocktail # 10
Date: 9/23/2002 12:44:22 P.M. Eastern Daylight Time
From: SLPGNP
To: Sharon's Med

Dear Loved Ones,

Chemo cocktail # 10. Choices—I am almost at the finish line of my chemo cocktails. I have learned so much in this race for the cure. I know I am supposed to drink fluids and exercise. Plenty of rest is always important, but how do I get emotionally healthy so I can cope with everything in my life without going to pieces? How can I keep from getting depressed? I think the answer is that you surround yourself with happy optimistic people who are really there for you. This may not be the time for you to solve the problems of the world. It is the time for you to soak in the good vibrations and let them surround you in love. I am looking toward the sunshine, the zoo, the museum, and to very kind people. I have simplified my life and am trying to be positive. Even when the nurse couldn't find a vein and I had to be jabbed three times, I tried to stay optimistic. You know the old adage, "Your cup is half empty or your cup is half full." I still choose full. Optimism isn't always easy to find when you are not well, but pessimism leads to despair. When I feel that way, I have to pick myself up, dust myself off, and start all over again. That is the only way. Giggle, laugh, smile, and think good thoughts. If that doesn't work, go get help. Clergy, a therapist, or a dear friend will sometimes be the antidote to bring you out of the blues. We all get down on ourselves even when we're healthy. Having cancer can make it tougher, but nothing is impossible because we're alive. Seek help, find an answer that you can be comfortable with. Plaster that smile on your beautiful face. I need to read this. Need to hear this. Like the little train trying to make it up the hill, "I know I can I know I can."

Love, Sharon

Subject: One More Mountain to Climb
Date: 10/9/2002 8:32:39 P.M. Eastern Daylight Time
From: SLPGNP
To: Cathlit

Dear Evelyn,

Ok, I may be black and blue but it is done. My veins just would not accept the mustard gas, (only kidding). It took four times. I decided I am so determined to get better I just didn't care. I finished at 1:38 A.M. I am so happy it is over. I barely sleep but I am not tired at night. I rode my bike 3½ miles at 5 A.M. Talk about clock confusion. My next one is October 21, God willing. I am going to be like a hermit until then.

Tomorrow I head back to the hospital for blood tests and Neupogen. I have a smile on my face and a glint in my eyes. My color is better. John brought over a juicer. I think I probably told you that. Well, this A.M. I had cantaloupe juice. It was very good. I also tried apple, carrot, celery, and parsley. Wow. That is an energy drink.

Much love, Sharon

Subject: Hurray! It's Over
Date: 10/24/2002 9:14:18 A.M. Eastern Daylight Time
From: SLPGNP
To: Sharon's Med

Dear Friends, Family, and Loved Ones,

It is Thursday morning and I am thrilled to report that the chemo is now over. I didn't get home until 2 A.M. Monday morning and was of course up all night trying to drink enough, to get it out of me. I broke out in hives on my chest. I guess it was the fond farewell from my body. My fingers swelled on my left hand, so I couldn't bend them. What it shows is each time you have chemotherapy the reaction may be different. My left leg, which is on the side where the chemo went in, turned purple. I think the veins were screaming "enough already." Today, the rash has all but faded and my leg is almost back to normal.

This has been quite a ride. I don't want this to happen to anyone ever, but at least I can say that I have gone through this in the most positive way I could.

I still have some more hills to climb, but hopefully the mountain summit has been reached. You have all helped me so much in spirit, hope, love, and encouragement. It is very scary to be told that you have two cancers and still put on a brave front. I can never thank you enough for all that you have done. You know exactly who you are and so does God, to whom I am very grateful.

Much love,
Sharon

Subject: Joy To The World
Date: 12/7/2002 12:29:53 A.M. Eastern Standard Time
From: SLPGNP
To: Sharon's Med

"Joy to the World" from Sharon, who is very grateful to be alive and well in Boca Raton. I can't believe I am home

after eight months, but here I am on December 7th. What an adventure I have had. You haven't heard from me lately because I got sick right before Thanksgiving and slept through that holiday.

George, "my prince," and I drove from Texas to Florida to relocate. We were so careful. However, just a few days in the Sunshine State brought out every flu bug known to man. I got it but good. I am happy to report that I am better as of today and moving forward once again.

It has been quite a journey from the day Evelyn put me, in tears, on the train in Charleston for a New York diagnosis of what was wrong with me. Who ever would have guessed? She drove to New York right after me, and we had some week, with all the tears, tests, and finally the trip to Texas.

Amy and John were there all the way. John took me by the hand and led me to M.D. Anderson, while Amy made babies "just for me." At this moment, I am waiting for Aaron, Amy, Amanda, and Andrea to arrive and see us.

It is 72 degrees, which is a lot better than zero in Jamesville. I feel truly blessed that I have such a fantastic family and superb friends, who are my sisters and brothers. Merry came to Houston twice to engineer the right chemo nurses for me. Thanks to her, my veins are intact.

The question of doing radiation came up and I was in quite a quandary for weeks. It was decided, however, to forgo it for now. The decision on what to do to prolong one's life can be overwhelming. I pray that the doctors and God are right there helping to guide me in the right direction.

Enjoy every day, and know how much I appreciate each and every one of you.

Anna came up from Bermuda and decided I needed more meditation and relaxation. What a good idea! We walked in the zoo. It was a great time. The animals are so smart. McCoy and McKenzie are particularly glad to be home. They headed right for the pool.

My dad looks about the same, and all of my mom's things are right where she left them. That gives me great comfort. There is a song called "There are Holes in the Floor of Heaven." I know my mom is watching me now.

Love you,
Sharon

Subject: (no subject)
Date: 2/27/2003 11:50:58 A.M. Eastern Standard Time
From: SLPGNP
To: Sharon's Med

Dear Everyone,

OK So I've been a delinquent. I thought everyone needed a break from all the news. Let's call it a holiday from cells and therapies. I have good news. I have been in Houston for the past three weeks having my first checkup since chemo 12. So far so good.

We are looking into the thyroid situation and although they see no growth, the doctor thinks it may still be there. We will deal with it as we go. Meanwhile, it is back to living a productive careful life. I am very grateful to be here and love being back in my home as a person on the right road to recovery.

Love you all,
Sharon

19

The Final Verdict

When you wish upon a star
makes no difference who you are
Anything your heart desires will come to you
from "When You Wish Upon a Star"

The countdown was coming ever closer, and after eight months in Houston, Texas, I would soon learn my fate. Had Dr. Goy been successful in eradicating the cancers from my body? Did I do everything in my power to follow his carefully laid out instructions aimed at a complete recovery? My instincts said, "Yes you have Sharon. You did it to the best of your ability." But was my best good enough?

The chemotherapies were all over and now, in just a few days, the final CT scans, sonograms, and PET scans would be done too. Then I'd see firsthand if the cancer cells had been eradicated. My mindset had been to "stomp on them," "squash them," and "send them to another planet," but now reality was setting in. I would soon learn the outcome.

My dear friend Anna Finkbeiner arrived in Houston for my final tests and scans because she had decided it would be the most meaningful time for the both of us. Hopefully the news would be positive and we could celebrate a victory together. She was bright, witty, and full of advice, given her English sense of propriety and her Bermuda style. Numerous times over the past thirty-five years, George and I had visited her on that quaint isle so isolated in the Atlantic. Now

130

she was visiting me far away from the harbors and tropical lifestyle.

It was a special time among friends. Chatting about a possible trip together made me feel exhilarated and optimistic about my future life, something I wanted desperately to hold onto. "How do I look," I asked my true friend, while walking through the zoo. It was the day before the scans were to begin.

"You look sensational, just like the giraffes over there," she replied, "considering what you have had to endure. Look at your energy level. I can hardly keep up with you girl!" I loved it when she called me "girl," a euphemism she often used to describe women of any age.

Anna made me laugh and feel good about myself. Even if it was not exactly true, the words she uttered were the perfect antidote for any uncertainty I might be feeling.

"Imagine a life free of cancer," I continued. "I would give anything just to hear those words."

"I think you will hear them," she reassured me. "You've followed Dr. Goy's program to the letter, and you seem fine to me, albeit with less hair on your head."

I laughed again. "I always wanted to get a perfect score in everything I've ever done, but this time I want it more than anything."

"Think positive." Anna replied quickly. "I think you are a winner this time."

That evening alone in my room, the "what ifs" slowly invaded my innermost thoughts. Could cancer cells still be multiplying in my body? The thoughts sent a chill down my spine and I decided to take a bath and wash my nearly bald head to focus on other issues.

- *Doing something constructive takes your mind off negative emotions that might be intent on disturbing your optimism.*

Bright and early the next morning, as George and I were sipping green tea in the kitchen, the phone rang. It was my sister-in-law, Sandy Richman calling from New York with her special message to cheer me on for the day ahead. "You are a most amazing person," she offered. "You are a coach for life. You find good in everything that happens and are able to turn it into a positive. Just keep it up!"

"Wow," I said. "No one ever put it quite like that. I love what you have told me. I'll keep these thoughts with me as a constant reminder."

- *Words of encouragement are necessary for cancer patients to hear, especially when the going gets rough and particularly on chemotherapy and testing days. Phone calls that lift the spirit and bring a smile are a welcome addition to every cancer patient's hope chest.*

With renewed confidence and a spring in my step, I knew that whatever challenges were in store for me that day, I was strong in spirit, mind, and heart and would meet them head-on. After today's tests, what I wanted to hear the most from Dr. Goy had now changed. I no longer wanted to hear, "You will be fine." Instead, the three most important words I could ever hear from him were "You *are* fine." Hopefully I would hear these words after all the testing was complete.

As Anna and I sat in the CT scan waiting room later that morning, I took a few moments to chat with my fellow patients who were still in the midst of their chemotherapy treatments. They were getting scans to see how their treatments were progressing. All my hopes and prayers were with them. We were one family now in our collective determination to beat the cancers.

I had survived everything thus far. I could still sing "Whistle a Happy Tune," look at the blue jay out the window, play "Around the World" on the piano, bake a carrot cake, teach English to the foreign-born, share my ideas on cancer, hug a grandchild, and let everyone who touched my life know how profoundly I appreciated everything they had done for me. I was one of the lucky ones because I was still here on this planet, still forging ahead and hoping for a bright future. Thinking about this gave me great comfort.

Before long, my name was called for my barium drink or "banana daiquiri." "Here's to life," I toasted as I clinked Anna's bottled water with a smile.

"Go for it girl," she answered brightly, as we walked around the M.D. Anderson Cancer Center to pass away the time. "I have a brilliant idea," she volunteered. "We'll have real banana daiquiris on my island as soon as you are able."

"I love your spirit and your plan," I tossed back at her. "One day I'll be there."

- *Accentuating the positive helps to defuse negative situations involving cancer therapy and makes it easier for the patient to focus on getting through whatever he or she needs to accomplish in a proactive and purposeful way.*

I had been poked, prodded, and scanned so many times over the previous eight months that this set of investigative scans seemed routine. Their outcome, however, was the most important of all and would tell me whether my future looked bright or bleak.

After three hours, the scans were over and I was free for the rest of the day. I went home and awaited the results and the words I longed to hear from Dr. Goy.

It didn't take long for the call to come, and the next morning we were back in the eighth floor waiting room of M.D. Anderson, awaiting the final verdict. Hand in hand, George and I walked into Dr. Goy's office with Anna by my side. George, trying to reassure me, whispered, "Don't worry, whatever the outcome, we will deal with it."

Dr. Goy was standing there in his long white coat with a broad smile on his face and a twinkle in his eyes. "You are fine," he said. "The scans show no sign of the cancer."

The words reverberated throughout my body. I was overwhelmed. I was filled with gratitude toward this brilliant doctor, who had told me eight months ago that two different cancers had invaded my body. Now he had accomplished everything that he said he would and that I hoped for, and done it while making me feel a part of the healing team. I was trembling. Tears of joy streamed down my face. I had a smile that wouldn't stop. George and Anna were hugging while Dr. Goy just stood there for a moment, reaping the rewards of his labor.

I looked at him and said, "I don't know where to begin to thank you for everything you have done for me. You have given me another chance at life and I am so grateful."

Smiling he said, "This is what I do. I like to see results like these. Beating cancer is a team effort, and we did it together. I'm giving you an A-plus for following all the directions."

I always liked to get an A and it was the perfect gift for him to give me.

Because so many others were in the waiting room hoping to hear the same words I had, I didn't want to take any more of his time. As we said our last goodbyes, Dr. Goy reminded me, "I'll see you again in twelve weeks. Meanwhile, drink plenty of fluids, eat sensibly, get your rest, and ride your exercise bike every day. Keep your positive attitude and get back to your normal life as soon as possible."

I would gladly follow his orders. I had my life back and would treasure it like a precious gift every day. Little things would no longer bother me, as I would try to focus on the bigger picture.

As we left Dr. Goy's office, I wanted to shout from the M.D. Anderson rooftops. "I'm a life lover. I have my life back. Thank you, thank you Dr. André Goy." But he wouldn't have heard me because he probably was already engrossed in figuring out how to save another patient's life. How lucky I was the day that Dr. Andy Zelenetz at Memorial Sloan-Kettering advised me to head west and find Dr. Goy. I heeded his advice. I found Dr. Goy. Now I could begin the rest of my life as a winner after all.

20

Approaching the Winner's Circle

The sun will come out, tomorrow
Bet your bottom dollar
That tomorrow, there'll be sun
Clears away the cobwebs and the sorrow
'Til there's none...

from "Tomorrow"

October 21, 2002

Time passes so quickly when you are busy moving in a positive direction. It doesn't matter what the focus is.

It's hard to believe that twelve chemotherapy sessions and eight months had flown by. Yes, there were days when I didn't feel well and cried out, "Why me?" but I hardly choose to remember those because they are relegated far into the background by all of the positive outcomes.

Think of it as delivering a baby. Memories of those intense labor pains fade quickly when you see your new, beautiful child. To me, cancer therapies are similar. It's the positive result we are all looking for.

I've always felt that God watched over me, even when I thought there was too much on my plate; but I never dreamed about what was going to land in my fifty-seven-year-old body. On the other hand, no one expects to be stricken with cancer; it just shows up like an uninvited guest.

It was a real shock to find out that I had additional, unrelated cancer cells that may have traveled from my thyroid gland to a lymph node in my chest. It had such a long name

I couldn't even pronounce it. I admit that at first, I cried in despair! Then I asked a lot of questions and never gave up despite exhaustion, hair loss, constipation, and periodic pain!

Part of the reason for my persistence was sheer determination and a need to seek answers, although they were not always easy to find. I desperately wanted to know why I had these cancers in two different parts of my body at the same time, but no one, not even the brilliant Dr. Goy, was able to tell me.

His focus was on the cure from the beginning; since I trusted him completely, I had to accept it and go forward.

When I wasn't feeling quite right, I didn't wait for the next appointment to ask questions; I called right away to seek help. I was a cancer neophyte after all. Now I'm much more knowledgeable and aware of the signs and the symptoms. Most people don't have a desire to learn about these illnesses, but when I did, I felt much less afraid and more in control.

- *In part, it was because of my confidence in Dr. Goy. He thought that my questions were relevant and therefore was always frank with his answers.*

I became an enthusiastic student of cancer. I felt free to ask and, by so doing, I absorbed the information like a damp sponge.

- *Relating well with your oncologist makes the whole experience that much easier.*

My family and friends are unreservedly supportive, and for that I feel truly blessed. My children and husband were diligent from the beginning, but then we've always been there for each other, through the good times and bad.

- *The people who really care about me make the cancers easier to endure by constant encouragement and love.*

Some came to visit, others called, and many sent cards during my stay away from home. I knew that I had a reason to live, love, fight, and go on!

- *No one should ever have to fight cancer alone. But if you do, speak up, and someone will come to assist you! Remember that most hospitals have either a volunteer program or patient advocates who are ready to help. Be sure to do your part and reach out.*

The volunteers and staff at M.D. Anderson and the Rotary House Marriott Hotel, across from the cancer center, where I often had a bite to eat and played the lobby piano, were so friendly and compassionate; it made such a difference to be treated like a normal person! I wanted desperately to be more than patient number 379421, a number I had to recite every time my blood was taken or a procedure performed.

I was a real person, with two serious diseases, who could cry just at the thought of my condition. The warmth and kindness shown by these total strangers was truly amazing! I know in my heart that it's one of the reasons I was able to conquer the enemy and concentrate on getting well.

Throughout my life, I always enjoyed being the giver, but now I had to learn to be a receiver as well. My passion to find a cancer cure has no bounds! I'm thrilled to be in remission. I hope to share my story with other "life lovers" who will listen, so that those who might be afraid to seek answers will gain the strength to go forward.

I used to have a difficult time even saying the word *cancer.* Now I face it squarely with the understanding that if I can, anyone can! I've learned so much, but I'm no longer frightened. I'll always attack cancer head-on, and I hope that anyone who is touched by it will remember the title of this book and have the courage to say, "Look Out Cancer...Here I Come!"

The Wind Beneath my Wings
It must have been cold there in my shadow,
To never have sunlight on your face?
You've been content to let me shine,
You always walked a step behind.

When you're lucky enough to have someone special in your life, it's important to show, by words and deeds, how much that person is appreciated. We've talked about how important your doctor is to a positive outcome, but your support system is also vital. If you don't have a husband or wife, you need a child, friend, or member of the clergy. You need someone who cares. Blend in some faith, joy, and optimism, and you'll be on the right road.

To recover from cancer, you need a reason to smile. Right now, I feel that I am among the most blessed persons on earth. People of every faith, color, and creed have shown their true feelings. I've been prayed for, written to, and visited. Receiving beautiful flowers, little gifts, and kind words has meant so much to building my spirit.

- *Go on! Move forward. You can beat this! You will beat this! That is the jump from maybe to absolutely, and you will make it too.*

- *When you have cancer, you quickly find out who really cares about you. I feel so lucky because I know.*

I don't really care where I live or what I have except for my family and friends. They are my most important treasures. If I learned one important thing, it is that nothing else really matters.

21

"Loving": The Long Road Home

Things look swell, Things look great
Gonna have the whole world on a plate,
Starting here, Starting now,
Honey, Ev'rything's coming up roses!
from "The Wind Beneath My Wings"

November 2002

Packed up and ready to go, George and I left Houston early one morning with McCoy and McKenzie, heading back to our home in Boca Raton, Florida. Saying good-bye to John, Chrissy, and the doctors wasn't easy, but knowing I was only a phone call away renewed my confidence.

Thirteen hundred miles is a long haul for anyone. I was so happy to be well enough to leave. It didn't matter how long the ride would be.

Chemotherapy had left its mark. My hair lay inside a velvet pillow next to me on the front seat. My fingers were still swollen from a drug reaction, and sometimes the toes on one of my feet felt numb. Even my derriere was shouting out with a fistula that appeared to have been due to constipation. The good news is that there are remedies for all of these maladies, time being one of them. Meanwhile, I sat on an inner tube in the car. It really works to alleviate pain on the underside.

Throughout life, your cup is half empty or half full. I always choose full. Optimism is an intangible that I believe in, and the kindness of God and humankind has never let me down.

Cancer is hard to conquer, but a positive attitude, along with caring and faith, helps pull you through.

Driving east on I-10 at more than seventy miles per hour was exhilarating. Together we would share anything and everything. Reminiscing about the past when we were young made us both smile. When I was twelve years old, I sang, "Have Faith, Hope and Charity," in front of the big grandstand in Rutland, at the Vermont State Fair. Ten thousand people filled the bleachers as Sharon Strauss, "the little girl from Danby with the big voice," sang her heart out. I was under contract to Jubilee Records and was often seen and heard on TV and radio in the Northeast, thrilled to be a little star in a big world.

Now, many years later, the song popped into my mind, and I realized that in order to lick cancer, you need to have faith, hope, and charity.

These three intangibles have been deeply ingrained in my personality for as long as I can remember. It's healthy for cancer patients and caregivers alike to look back and remember the good times. It will bring a smile to your face. We all know that's a good thing.

Baton Rouge was just down the road where we would stop for our first night's rest. Everywhere I looked, there was beauty to behold. It was a privilege to be alive and I knew it.

"It's almost Thanksgiving and I can't believe I'll be home to enjoy it," I said with a big smile.

"You've come through this with flying colors, and I'm so proud of you," George replied enthusiastically. "You're an amazing woman!"

Those positive words resound in my head over and over. It's the "pill" I need to keep going forward. It's the kind of praise that we all need to hear.

"Am I imagining things or did the time in Houston fly?" I asked him with a lilt in my voice.

"You're imagining things, but you were on a schedule and followed it perfectly, concentrating so hard on getting it right the first time. I don't think you were worrying about what month it was."

I couldn't have agreed more.

"Pinch yourself," I said, aloud, as I gently squeezed my arm. "I'm so lucky to be going home and getting a second chance."

As we pulled into the Residence Inn, the thought of 9/11 flashed through my mind again. How I remembered heading south on I-95 that fateful day, from Charleston, South Carolina, to Boca Raton, my ears riveted to the radio. Now, we were on I-10, heading to the same place. I was facing a new beginning, having been given a second chance; I thought of all the people who weren't so lucky.

Back on the road early the next morning, I was thinking about what I could do to help another person get rid of cancer. I thought about Dr. Goy's final remarks. "We want you healthy and growing stronger every day. You'll come back in three months for a checkup," He told me. I knew what that meant: more sonograms, CT scans and blood tests. They would continue at intervals as a part of my life, but I still had it: life. It was still in me, and I loved the feeling.

I would continue to see Dr. Goy wherever he was. I would want this expert to tell me that the cancer had disappeared. That is the dream of every cancer patient.

"I'm a life lover," I said to George with a big smile. We were now past Mobile, Alabama.

"You always come up with these sayings."

"I know," I said softly. "It just happens."

"Here's to life and to our future," he said, pretending to hold a drink, as he drove toward Pensacola. We clinked "glasses" in the air.

"Delicious," I said, "let's make plans for the future."

"Now, that's what I like to hear," he replied.

"Our house," I said, "What kind of condition do you think it's in?"

"After almost a year of not living there, I'm sure there's plenty to do," he answered with a smile.

"I'm already thinking of making a few changes," I declared optimistically.

"Not so fast," he cautioned. "Priorities for you include: rest, exercise, water, meditation, smiling, singing, playing the piano, and eating healthful foods."

"I know you're right, but there's always the Home and Garden Channel to watch."

"That will be fine. We'll roll like the ocean waves and tackle what we need to, leaving the rest for another day."

I wanted to do everything, but he had the right idea. Take baby steps and love every day on this earth. God was very good to me. He needed me right here with George and my setters, McCoy and McKenzie, my family, and my friends.

Perhaps, sharing my story with all who would listen and maybe making a difference in someone's life, would be the greatest reward I could ever have.

"I'm going to do it," I said aloud. "My hand is outstretched, just waiting to touch someone."

"To tomorrow and a bright new future," George said.

"I just love the sound of that. Let's go home and love every minute of the ride," was my reply.

22

Nothing Ventured, Nothing Gained...

You got to try a little kindness
Yes show a little kindness
Just shine your light for everyone to see
from "Everything's Coming Up Roses"

It was time for my six-month checkup to determine whether my upper chest and other potential tumor sites were clean, with no sign of infiltrates. I felt a sense of excitement and a bit of apprehension as I once again boarded a plane that would take me this time, to Hackensack, New Jersey, instead of Houston, Texas, for my CT scans. I'd also be seen by the doctor who'd given me the right combination of drugs and an attitude that hopefully chewed those cancer cells into oblivion.

I wasn't overly surprised when I heard that Dr. André Goy was leaving M.D. Anderson to become the Chief of Lymphoma at Hackensack University Medical Center; a rapidly growing cancer center in the Northeast.

Every time I saw him for my biweekly chemotherapy checkups in Texas, Dr. Goy was full of life—excited about the research he was doing—yet always the consummate clinician. "I don't know how he does it," I'd often remark to George on my return to our rented townhouse in Houston. "He's so positive and committed to finding new therapies for cancer."

"I notice it myself," George would reply. "His enthusiasm makes everyone he comes in contact with less afraid and more determined to help in his search for a cure."

By now, I was strong in my heart and my soul. I knew that I was one of the lucky ones to have been placed in Dr. Goy's care. And as long as I was able, I'd find a way to follow him, wherever he might be saving lives.

- *I still wanted the doctor who tried to make all of his patients feel they were part of the cure. It didn't matter where.*

A plane ride was now an option for me, although I had a carbon face mask in my purse just in case people were coughing too much on the aircraft. It was my way of protecting myself if I thought it necessary. My white blood cell count had rebounded to normal levels and I was confident that "I'd be fine" as I boarded Spirit Airlines, bound for LaGuardia Airport in New York.

It was the first week of March, and the warm breezes of South Florida were already flowing in, giving us just a hint of the hot summer ahead. I brought along a fur-lined coat I had saved from my former northern life, just in case the chill in the Northeast still lingered.

George had made my reservation on a no-frills airline and was able to get me a bulkhead seat on just two days notice. In only three hours, I'd hopefully be driving over the George Washington Bridge in a rental car that had been reserved at LaGuardia Airport. I'd never driven to Hackensack University Medical Center but knew from the directions that it was just a stone's throw from the George Washington Bridge.

As I sat in my window seat, I was fingering my mask. Should I put it on and scare everyone walking by me? I have learned from experience that people don't realize that when someone wears a mask, it's because of concern about his or her own health issues. Very low white blood cell counts can mean trouble for anyone who comes in contact with a serious infection while undergoing chemotherapy. This was no longer my concern. I knew that I was better, but the thought still lingered, "What if? What if?" as I played with the elastic strap on the mask.

A well-dressed middle-aged man sat down next to me. "He must be going to a meeting," I thought to myself as I watched him opening his laptop.

We greeted each other casually, as I fastened my seat belt. It didn't take long for him to spot the mask. At first he didn't say a word, seemingly preoccupied with the information on his computer. As we prepared for takeoff, it was obvious that flying was second nature to him, and he didn't seem to notice the stewardess giving emergency instructions.

"Excuse me," he asked inquisitively, "Why the mask?" That was my cue I thought, as we were climbing to our cruising altitude of thirty-one thousand feet.

I quickly recounted what had happened to me, how I had been misdiagnosed with allergies in South Carolina and had come to New York for an accurate diagnosis. Then it was off to Houston, Texas, to be cured of what was really ailing me. The mask was my protective shield whenever I flew, even if I no longer needed it. Now, I was going to Hackensack, New Jersey, following the outstanding oncologist who I was confident would be a leading force in figuring out how to eradicate the disease that had invaded my body.

"What do you do?" I heard myself asking my new traveling companion.

"I'm a professional fund raiser for foundations."

The words that he uttered resounded in my head. I had just finished writing a book that would help many others afflicted with lymphoma and was starting the Life Lover™ Foundation, intended to let all the profits from my book go to new and novel therapies that held promise for a cure.

It was my belief, and the notion that gave me the fortitude to go on, that a higher authority had decided that I would be stricken, made well again and enabled to spread the word through a book and foundation. I felt that we can all play a role in finding the cure, whether we have medical backgrounds or not. Perhaps God had deliberately seated this man with a wealth of foundation and fund-raising expertise next to me. He, in turn, would commit to becoming a partner in convincing those who were interested that we were on a serious mission. I pledged that if I were able, I would spend the rest of my life supporting the research, development, and therapies of Dr. André Goy and others who were on a mission to end cancer.

The time passed quickly as we shared ideas. I had little time to notice that the sky had turned from vivid blue to a drab gray and that the rain and snow was pelting the windows. "Ladies and gentlemen, please fasten your seatbelts," I vaguely heard the captain say. "We're heading into some rough weather ahead and the airports in the New York area are shutting down. We still have permission to land, with alternatives at Washington, D.C., Philadelphia, and Wilmington, Delaware."

Ordinarily, this would have caused concern, but somehow the news didn't faze me. I was sitting next to an experienced fundraiser who heard my story and said, "I'm going to help you. Have you ever started a foundation before?"

"No, I haven't," I had to admit, "but I've learned over the past few years that more money is needed for cancer research. That is why the Life Lover™ Foundation was born." Over the months of trying to be optimistic about the future, I had often said to anyone who would listen, "I'm a life lover; I don't want to die."

I also had Dr. Goy's phrase at the back of my mind, *"You'll be fine. You'll be fine."* Call it the repayment plan, but I didn't want anyone else to go through the torment of thinking that his or her life might be over because of a diagnosis of cancer. Knowing the brilliant researcher who was on the cutting edge of the latest theories was the first part of the equation. I had a serious fundraiser seated right next to me, and I was the patient who could share with the world the best way to get through it all and come out with a full life. The formula was now complete. We'd be winners after all.

I barely felt the landing gear go down as we were finally allowed to land at LaGuardia, in a blinding snow squall one hour behind schedule. What a skilled pilot, I thought, as we used the entire runway before making the turn toward the terminal. There was not another plane in sight as we headed into the freezing cold, but I didn't care. I was safely wrapped in my warm winter coat, with a new ally on my side willing to join me and many others who would work together to make cancer a thing of the past.

"Remember polio," he said, as we waved good-bye.

"I forgot about polio," I replied, and "hopefully lymphoma and other cancers will soon be in the same category."

Coming to Hackensack University Medical Center in the Northeast was a big leap from M.D. Anderson in the Southwest. But since it was Dr. Goy's decision to join a promising cancer center to further develop his interest in clinical trials and cancer research, I had confidence and a strong belief that brilliant minds attract each other, no matter where they are.

It didn't take long for me to discover that other prominent clinicians and cancer researchers were also coming from across the country from as far away as the Fred Hutchinson Cancer Center in Seattle; the Mayo Clinic in Rochester, Minnesota; Johns Hopkins University in Baltimore, Maryland; the Myeloma Center in Little Rock, Arkansas; Memorial Sloan-Kettering in New York; as well as M.D. Anderson in Houston, Texas.

From everything I have learned on this road to wellness, one idea stands out: If you have good communication and confidence in your doctor and he or she has successful results in treating your disease, then this is the oncologist to choose to continue with no matter where his or her medical career might go.

The question then comes up as to whether it is economically feasible, practical, or logistically possible to go to a different location for checkups or treatment. For some patients the answer is "I simply can't." However, there is a great opportunity to stay in touch with those oncologists who have treated you or advised you along the way. I have found that they are eager to know about your progress and may answer questions or concerns you have by either telephone or the Internet. In fact, every oncologist and physician who helped me on this journey is excited and pleased with the outcome.

It's what Dr. Goy said to me with a broad smile that final day in Houston when I thanked him so much for all of his efforts. It remains emblazoned in my memory, reminding me to think positive thoughts and move forward with my life.

"This is what it is about," he stated, looking straight into my eyes, "and these are the results I like to see. Remember, beating cancer is a team effort and we did it together."

Dr. Goy can be reached at the Cancer Center at HUMC in Hackensack, New Jersey. Their web site is www.humc.com.

Tips for Feeling Better—
Inside and Out

- Try to start the day with a smile; it's great to be alive.
- Hope is the intangible that lets the sunshine into your mind and spirit.
- Laugh, laugh, and laugh some more; it's a healthy thing to do.
- Sing happy songs, play music, dance, do anything that lifts your spirit.
- Remember to think happy thoughts.
- Exercise on a stationary bike or walk as much as you can.
- Drink plenty of fresh water as well as green and black tea.
- Love up your dogs or an animal, stuffed or real.
- Tell those who love you how much you love them each and every day.
- Remember that kind words, thoughts, and deeds can work miracles for everyone.

Glossary

It was almost as if I had landed on another planet when Hodgkin's lymphoma and thyroid cancer came into my life. A whole new world of words were being thrown at me, and to be honest, I didn't have a clue what they meant. Oh, I had heard some of them before, but I was never concerned enough to learn their significance. I needed to write down the meanings so that I could go back and figure out just exactly what the doctors and nurses were talking about. The following definitions are compiled from various authoritative medical sources.

ABVD—Adriamycin, bleomycin, vinblastine, and dacarbazine are four of the drugs used in Hodgkin's lymphoma chemotherapy.

Benign tumor—A swelling or growth that is not cancerous (not malignant).

Biopsy—A medical procedure whereby a piece of tissue or fluid is taken from one's body and examined with a microscope and/or other device to determine whether or not the tissues are normal.

Cancer—An abnormal uncontrollable proliferation of cells.

Carcinogen—A substance or agent known (or strongly suspected) to cause cancer.

CT (computed tomography) Scan—A diagnostic test that uses both x-rays and a computer to create a two- or three-dimensional picture of your head, chest, abdo-

men, pelvis, or extremities. It is used to detect disease
or abnormal structures in organs.

Chemotherapy—Treatment with anticancer, chemically
based medicines. Many times, these powerful drugs are
injected into your arm or through a portal placed in
your chest.

Dexamethasone (Decadron)—A synthetic corticosteroid
that makes the side effect of chemotherapy bearable by
decreasing nausea, it is also used widely in the treatment of lymphoma as an anti-tumor agent but also
used for pain control (reduces inflammation and swelling).

Echocardiogram—A diagnostic test that evaluates the size
and function of the heart. It is a painless test based on
ultrasound.

Fine needle aspiration—A procedure that assesses a lump
using a syringe and needle whereby saline is flushed
into and back out of the suspect tissue to capture its
loose cells. FNA is an alternative to a surgical biopsy. It
is a simple procedure that can provide information to
your doctor regarding whether a tissue mass or cyst is
benign or malignant.

Granulomas—Small inflammatory nodules that form in the
affected tissue. Granulomas are groups of immune cells
that are normally a part of the body's defense system.

Helicobacter pylori—A bacteria that survives in the stomach and can cause gastric ulcers, stomach cancer or
lymphoma.

Hodgkin's disease—A type of lymphoma that has a different cell structure than non-Hodgkin's lymphoma and is
characterized by Reed-Sternberg cells, named for the
doctors who initially described these cells. It is thought
that B lymphocytes, or antibody-producing white cells,
are mutated becoming unable to function normally.
They then become malignant and multiply, no longer
regulated by normal biofeedback mechanisms. Hodg-

kin's lymphoma spreads in a contiguous manner, from node to nearby node.

Malignant tumor—A tumor that is cancerous, grows uncontrollably, and metastasizes (travels) to locations elsewhere in the body.

Meningioma—A benign tumor that develops in the thin membrane, or meninges, that covers the brain and spinal cord. They usually grow slowly and do not invade surrounding normal tissue and they rarely spread to other parts of the central nervous system or body.

MRI (magnetic resonance imaging)—A diagnostic test that uses magnetic field induced changes in tissues to create three-dimensional computerized images of the brain, spine, bones, and soft tissues of the body.

Non-Hodgkin's lymphoma—Cancer of the immune system which spreads more rapidly than Hodgkin's disease systemically outside the lymph nodes.

Neupogen (filgrastim)—A drug used to help chemotherapy patients rebuild their white blood cell counts to fight possible infections.

Oncology—The study and treatment of cancer.

PET (positron emission tomography) scan—A technology based on metabolic differences between normal and tumor tissues using radioactive glucose. In addition to CAT scan (which gives an idea of volumetric changes such as enlarged lymph nodes). PET scan gives an idea of the activity of the tumor and is also called functional imaging.

Phlebotomist—A trained practitioner who collects blood samples and body fluids from patients for laboratory testing.

Port(al)—A catheter placed in a vein to receive medication.

Procrit (epoetin alfa)—A drug used to help anemic chemotherapy patients rebuild red blood cells and thereby improve oxygen exchange and overall strength.

Radiation therapy—x-ray treatment that damages or kills cells. Lymphoma patients often receive a combination of chemotherapy and radiation or only one therapeutic modality, depending on the individual case.

Red blood cells—Cells that bring oxygen to tissues and take carbon dioxide away from them. During chemotherapy, these cells can be affected adversely; medication may be required to boost their production.

Remission—The disappearance of all cancer-related symptoms or findings.

Saline solution—A solution of sodium chloride and distilled water used to dilute chemotherapy or antibiotics.

Sarcoidosis—A disease of unknown cause that leads to inflammation in the lymph nodes, lungs, liver, eyes, skin, and/or other tissues.

SED rate (sedimentation rate)—The rate at which red blood cells settle down in a tube of blood under standard conditions; a high rate usually indicates the presence of inflammation somewhere in the body.

Side effects—Problems that occur when treatment affects healthy cells. Common side effects of cancer treatments can include fatigue, nausea, vomiting, decreased blood cell counts, hair loss and mouth sores. Many of these effects can be greatly reduced by medications and by following specific directions from the medical team.

Surgical Oncologist—A doctor who specializes in cancer surgery.

Tumor—Cells that group together and keep growing and crowding out normal cells. A tumor can be benign (not cancer) or malignant (cancer).

White blood cells—A general term for a variety of cells whose job is to fight invading bacteria, viruses, fungi, other infectious entities and allergy-causing agents.

Ultrasound—A diagnostic tool using sound waves to create an echo pattern that reveals the structures of organs and tissues.

Glossary

Vesicant—As related to chemotherapy, a strong drug that enters the vein and can cause tissue damage if it leaks or spreads outside the veins.

Web sites for cancer information:

www.ncbi.nlm.nih.gov/entrez/query.fcgi

www.cancersociety.com

www.cancerlinksusa.com/throid/nic_physician.htm

www.webmd.com

www.leukimia.org/hm_lls

www.lymphomafoundation.org

www.clinicaltrials.gov

www.asco.org/

www.hematology.org

www.lrf.org.uk/

Products that Improved
My Quality of Life

100% aloe vera gel—This light and cool gel made my skin feel so good. I'd just dab it on my cheeks or hands.

Biotene—antibacterial mouthwash and toothpaste. This fabulous product helped me through chemotherapy. I rinsed my mouth with the very gentle and pleasant-tasting mouthwash after each meal and before bed. I used the toothpaste at least three times a day. The result was healthy gums, strong teeth, and no mouth problems during my treatment. These are available at Costco, Walgreen's, Wal-Mart, and Randall's.

Disinfectant wipes—Some supermarkets and gas stations are providing their customers disinfectant wipes for use on the cart and pump handles.

Exertec stationary bike—I tried to ride several miles every day. This bike enabled me to move my arms as well as my legs.

Olive Oil—A healthy alternative to butter. A capful in the bath water improved my skin.

Organic shampoo 365—I not only ate organically grown fruits and vegetables, but I tried to use products with fewer chemicals.

Organically grown fruits and vegetables—Pesticides can contribute to causing certain cancers. I learned to avoid them whenever possible.

Patsy's all natural pasta sauces—No cholesterol or added sugar. When I wanted a taste of Italy, a spoon of a healthy tomato sauce over my pasta was the answer. Only fresh ingredients are ever used in Patsy's sauces—sweet peppers, mushrooms, and a touch of garlic worked for me. (Available at Rice Epicurean, Publics, and Randall's Flagship stores. www.patsys.com or 1.800.3patsys)

Purified or ozonated bottled water—Walgreen's, Eckerd, or any favorite brand of half-liter (500-mL) bottles. I drank it right from the bottle and found it easier to consume more that way.

Soy Delicious frozen desserts—A terrific alternative if digesting fats is a problem. A nondairy frozen dessert that is fruit-sweetened. My secret was a spoon of Vermont maple syrup and a handful of blueberries or sliced bananas on top—Yum. (Purchased at Whole Foods Market and produced by Turtle Mountain, Inc., Junction City, OR)

Spectrum Naturals grape seed oil. No *trans*-fatty acids, light-tasting, polyunsaturated oil. Perfect for sautéing, salads, soups, or baking. Sometimes I dabbed it on my hands or feet. It's very soft and gentle. (Available at Whole Foods Markets or Spectrum Organic Products, Inc., Petaluma, CA)

The Hope Rose

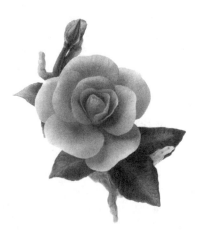

This magnificent Hope Rose is being offered to those who wish to support the Life Lover™ Foundation, Inc.

It's made by the Boehm Porcelain Company www.boehmporcelain.com.

I became acquainted with Boehm porcelains many years ago in my mother's antique shop in Vermont. I learned of their value as collectors from all over the world sought them out. I appreciated their intrinsic beauty at a very young age.

When our family moved to the beautiful village of Tuxedo Park, New York, twenty-five years ago, I became a member of the Tuxedo Park Garden Club. During my first year as a member, the club held a fundraiser. The grand prize was a Boehm porcelain bird and flower. I remember buying twenty chances hoping I might win. Sure enough I did! I've been a collector ever since.

When I was first diagnosed with cancer in April 2002, I learned that changing the old stagnant water from fresh flowers might be unhealthy to a person whose immune system is compromised while undergoing chemotherapy. Although fresh flowers are very beautiful, the water in the vase becomes full of bacteria—not at all good for a compromised immune system.

The answer was clear as a bell. I asked my husband, George, if he would bring a few of my Boehm flowers to Houston, where I was being treated. He granted my wish, and every day I had a Boehm rose in my bedroom and another beautiful flower in the living room. These handmade beauties will live on forever and become heirlooms that can be passed on for generations.

I am thrilled that Boehm porcelain has agreed, because of my cancer story, to produce a limited edition of the magnificent flower called the Hope Rose. A portion of the price of this hand-made collectors' edition will go to the Life Lover™ Foundation, Inc., under the medical direction of Dr. André Goy. This outstanding lymphoma and Hodgkin's disease research specialist named the rose and gave me the inspiration and hope I needed to beat this potential killer. It is from humankind's generosity that we will find a cure for these diseases, which combined, strike more than two hundred thousand people each year in America as well as in Western Europe.

"I'm A Life Lover™" Necklace

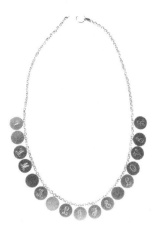

This beautiful necklace has been created by Concord Jewelers, a division of Hammerman Bros.

I was eighteen years old when I received my first piece of Hammerman Brothers jewelry. This designer and manufacturer of fine rings, bracelets, pins, necklaces, and earrings was then located on 58th Street in New York City.

George Parker, nineteen years old at the time, was meeting me in Manhattan and we were having dinner with his parents later that evening at the Concord Hotel at Kiamesha Lake, New York. Waiting outside in front of Joe Platt's garage on West 48th Street, I remember glancing at my watch and wondering how we were going to make the ninety-mile trip in less than two hours, when George appeared in a shiny white convertible. He had a big smile on his face as he pulled in and reached over to open the door. I hopped right into my seat saying a quick good-bye to Mr. Platt, who not only owned the parking lot but was also a Concord Hotel guest.

George wasted no time in pulling from his pocket a small black leather box and saying, "This is for you." Quickly opening it, I saw a beautiful diamond engagement ring. I couldn't believe it, right in broad daylight on 48th Street, I got engaged. The ring was from Hammerman Bros.

Forty years later, while I was still wearing the same beautiful ring, Robert, Darcy, and Brett Hammerman, now located on 57th Street, presented me with a 14 karat gold necklace for the Life Lover™ Foundation. This ray of hope, which beautifully spells out "I'm A Life Lover," will be awarded to those people who contribute to finding a cure for these cancers through foundation giving. I uttered this phrase many times when I needed spirit and hope. Wearing it makes me feel happy and grateful to be alive.

About the Author

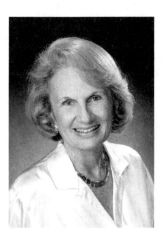

Sharon Parker is the Founding Director of the Life Lover™ Foundation, a philanthropic organization devoted to funding today's molecular research for tomorrow's cancer cures. With a masters degree in gerontology, she has served as an adjunct professor at the University of Northern Colorado's Graduate School of Gerontology and as the director of the nationally distinguished Retired Senior Volunteer Program in Boulder County, Colorado.

Sharon has also worked for Action, the Government volunteer agency. Her program was used as a model for the set up of other RSVP's across the country. While serving as director of the Volunteer and Information Center for Boulder County, Colorado, she brought the program to new levels of excellence and national recognition. At Colorado University, she taught an accredited course on volunteer management, a program sponsored by the United Way of America. She was also the director of the Braille Institute of America program for the blind and visually impaired elderly in Palm Beach County, Florida.

Sharon is also an extensive experience as an entertainer and as a leading figure in the resort industry. She was a professional actress and singer, starting at the age of ten.

She first appeared on television with Paul Winchell and Jerry Mahoney on ABC. Jubilee Records produced her first single, *Matching Kisses*. Sharon recorded for ABC Paramount and had a hit-of-the-week with *Don't let Him Know* when she was eighteen. Interviewed on both radio and television, Sharon's popularity grew and she performed at many clubs including The Concord, Grossinger's, Kutchers, Nevele, and at the Hotel Taft with Vincent Lopez. Once married to George Parker, of the legendary Concord Resort Hotel, Sharon quickly established herself as an institution at the hotel. As an official hostess to the stars, Sharon welcomed singers and comedians as well as those attending conventions at the hotel, which often had three thousand guests in the Concord dining room on Saturday nights.

Also while at the Concord, Sharon gave talks about the history of the Concord; she wrote the Concord's weekly contribution to the "Round the Resorts" section for the *New York Post* for many years.

Sharon Parker can be reached through her Website: www.lifeloverfoundation.org.

If you wish to support research for molecular cancer research, please send donations to:

Life Lover Foundation, Inc.
P.O. Box 881154
Boca Raton, FL 33488

Consumer Health Titles
from Addicus Books
Visit our online catalog at www.AddicusBooks.com

The Surgery Handbook—A Guide to Understanding
Your Operation $14.95
Understanding Lumpectomy—A Treatment Guide
for Breast Cancer $14.95
Understanding Parkinson's Disease—
A Self-Help Guide $14.95
Understanding Your Living Will $12.95
Your Complete Guide to Breast Augmentation
& Body Contouring $21.95
Your Complete Guide to Breast Reduction
& Breast Lifts $21.95
Your Complete Guide to Facial Cosmetic Surgery. . . . $19.95
Your Complete Guide to Face Lifts. $21.95
Your Complete Guide to Nose Reshaping $21.95

Organizations, associations, corporations, hospitals, and other groups may qualify for special discounts when ordering more than 24 copies. For more information, please contact the Special Sales Department at Addicus Books. Phone (402) 330-7493.

Email: info@AddicusBooks.com

Please send:

_____copies of_____

(*Title of book*)

at $ _____each   TOTAL: _____

Nebraska residents add 6% sales tax   _____

Shipping/Handling
  $4.00 postage for first book.
  $1.10 postage for each additional book   _____

          TOTAL ENCLOSED: _____

Name_____

Address _____

City _____State _____Zip _____

☐ Visa   ☐ MasterCard   ☐ American Express

Credit card number_____Expiration date _____

Order by credit card, personal check or money order.
Send to:

Addicus Books
Mail Order Dept.
P.O. Box 45327
Omaha, NE 68145
Or, order TOLL FREE: 800-352-2873
or online at
www.AddicusBooks.com